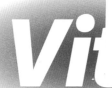

# COPD

*Your essential reference for the management
of Chronic Obstructive Pulmonary Disease
in primary care*

### Rachel Booker

*COPD Module Leader,
Education for Health, Warwick;
Member of the British Thoracic Society
COPD Consortium*

**CLASS HEALTH · LONDON**

*Printing history*
First published 2005
Reprinted 2006

The author and publishers welcome feedback from the users of this book.
Please contact the publishers.
**Class Publishing, Barb House,
Barb Mews, London W6 7PA, UK
Telephone: 020 7371 2119
Fax: 020 7371 2878 [International +4420]
Email: post@class.co.uk
Website: www.class.co.uk**

A CIP catalogue for this book is available from the British Library

ISBN 1 85959 114 0

Edited by Richenda Milton-Thompson

Designed and typeset by Martin Bristow

Printed and bound in Slovenia by Delo Tiskarna
by arrangement with Korotan, Ljubljana

### Acknowledgements
With thanks to my colleagues at Education for Health for their unfailing support
and encouragement, my numerous clinical colleagues and friends, particularly
David Bellamy, Jon Miles and June Roberts, for their words of wisdom and
enlightenment, and my family for their support, tolerance and forbearance
of my periods of distraction and the time I spend away from them.

# Contents

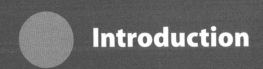

# Introduction

*Dear Colleagues*

## Welcome to *Vital COPD*

This practical book is designed for you to use during your work in general practice and the community, to enable you to deliver the best possible care to your patients with chronic obstructive pulmonary disease (COPD). COPD is a relatively new term for an old problem; variously described as 'chronic bronchitis', emphysema and chronic obstructive airways disease (COAD).

The book gives you the vital information you need to diagnose and manage this important, disabling condition. The detailed **contents list** allows you to pinpoint specific topics easily. The text is divided into ten distinct **chapters** with topics clearly presented. At the end of each topic you will find one or more **vital points** that will give you the essential information in a few key words. At the end of most chapters you will find an associated section called **patient and carer information**. These pages can be enlarged and photocopied for your patients.

You will find useful addresses and contact numbers at the end of the book, as well as references and further reading and details of training courses. There is also a **feedback form** on page 111, which I hope you will use. I would welcome comments and suggestions for improvements.

I hope that you will find this book useful, time-saving and vital to your everyday clinical practice and that, in using it, you will be able to provide an up-to-date and consistent standard and quality of health care for people with COPD.

*Rachel Booker*

# 1 COPD: Definition and impact

*'Chronic obstructive pulmonary disease (COPD) is characterised by airflow obstruction. The airflow obstruction is usually progressive, not fully reversible and does not change markedly over several months. The disease is predominantly caused by smoking.'* (NICE 2004)

COPD is the internationally recognised term for what was previously known as:

- Chronic bronchitis and emphysema
- Chronic obstructive airways disease (COAD)
- Chronic airflow limitation (CAL)
- Chronic obstructive lung disease (COLD)
- Chronic airflow obstruction (CAO)

## CAUSES

- Cigarette smoking is, overwhelmingly, the most important cause of COPD, accounting for around 90% of cases in the UK. Although COPD can occur in people who have never smoked, this is unusual
- 15–20% of smokers are susceptible to COPD and will experience an accelerated decline in their lung function as a direct result of smoking
- Susceptible smokers lose lung function at twice (or more) the normal rate. The more cigarettes they smoke, the more rapid their loss of lung function will be
- Smoking cessation will reduce the rate of lung function decline to that of a non-smoker or non-susceptible smoker. Lost lung function cannot be regained, but worthwhile salvage of lung function and improvement in life expectancy can be expected at any stage of the disease
- The earlier a susceptible smoker stops the better

Other risk factors include:

- Low birth weight
- Recurrent lower respiratory tract infection in childhood
- Low socioeconomic status
- Occupational exposure to high concentrations of organic and inorganic dusts, fumes and solvents (eg mining, welding)
- Genetic/familial susceptibility
- Alpha 1 antitrypsin deficiency

- These other risk factors generally increase an individual's susceptibility to cigarettes rather than cause clinically significant COPD on their own. As a general rule they should be considered as additive to the detrimental effects of smoking in a susceptible individual
- Some people with asthma develop a degree of irreversible airflow obstruction, either as a result of their asthma, particularly if they have not been treated adequately with inhaled corticosteroids, or because they have also smoked

## PATHOLOGY

The term COPD encompasses a mixture of disease processes:

- Chronic bronchitis and small airway disease (chronic bronchiolitis)
- Emphysema
- Some cases of chronic asthma
- The composition of this mixture varies between individuals. Some will have predominant emphysema, some chronic bronchitis. In practice most will have a combination of the first two but, where asthma predominates, the individual is likely to have more reversible disease and a better response to therapy

As COPD progresses, disruption of gas exchange can result in chronic hypoxia and cor pulmonale.

### Chronic bronchitis and small airway disease

*'Chronic bronchitis is the production of phlegm (sputum) on most days for three months during any two consecutive years'* (MRC 1965)

- While not all smokers with chronic bronchitis develop the airflow obstruction that characterises COPD, chronic cough and sputum is a significant symptom:
  - 18% of all smokers aged over 35 will have airflow obstruction
  - 27% of all smokers aged over 35 and with chronic cough will have airflow obstruction
  - 48% of all smokers aged over 60 and with chronic cough will have airflow obstruction
- Small airway disease, which affects airways less than 2–3 mm in diameter, is often associated with chronic bronchitis
- Major, irreversible structural changes can occur without causing symptoms. Generally, patients only present with breathlessness when damage is advanced
- The structural changes that result in irreversible airway narrowing and distortion are:
  - Inflammation
  - Thickening of the muscle layer
  - Oedema of the airway wall
  - Fibrosis around the airway
  - Mucus plugging

## Emphysema

- Emphysema is a destructive process involving the alveoli and, in its severe form, the terminal bronchioles and alveolar ducts as well
- Destruction of alveolar walls reduces the surface area of the lung, and impairs exchange of oxygen and carbon dioxide. This leads to abnormal blood gas levels
- Loss of alveolar tissue reduces the natural elasticity of the lungs. Exhalation becomes less efficient, resulting in over-inflation of the lungs
- The natural elasticity of alveolar walls provides support for small airways. When this is lost the small airways tend to collapse during exhalation, resulting in airflow obstruction and air trapping

## Asthma

- Asthma can result in fixed airflow obstruction as a result of:
  - Collagen deposition in the walls of the airways
  - Smooth muscle hypertrophy
  - Oedema
- 10% of people with childhood onset asthma and 25% of those with adult onset asthma will develop some degree of fixed airflow obstruction
- Asthmatics who smoke are more likely to develop fixed airflow obstruction
- Appropriate use of inhaled corticosteroids may reduce the risk

## Cor pulmonale

Chronic hypoxia eventually leads to complications involving the heart. By mechanisms that are still not fully understood chronic hypoxia leads to:

- Secondary polycythaemia
- Pulmonary hypertension
- Fluid retention and oedema
- Right ventricular strain and hypertrophy. Eventually the right ventricle will fail, leading to further oedema

## IMPACT OF COPD

- COPD is a common problem, often undiagnosed in the early stages (there are 900,000 diagnosed cases in the UK, but the true figure is likely to be nearer 1.5 million)
- COPD results in 30,000 premature deaths a year
- One in 8 emergency medical admissions to hospital are for COPD; patients utilise a large proportion of primary and secondary health care resources
- Cost to the health service is around £100,000,000 annually
- Costs to society are also high. Nearly 22 million working days are lost every year due to COPD

### The impact on patients

- COPD is a disabling condition. Slowly progressive breathlessness prevents patients from carrying out normal daily activities such as shopping and housework and may eventually make washing and dressing difficult
- Increasing breathlessness and disability produces psychosocial consequences:
  - Loss of confidence
  - Loss of role and self esteem
  - Increased dependency
  - Social isolation
  - Anxiety and depression

## The impact on families and carers

- Inability to work or forced early retirement may produce financial hardship
- Progressive disability will disrupt retirement plans and increase the burden of care on relatives and carers
- Relatives and carers can also become anxious and depressed

### VITAL POINT

*✳ Although COPD is slowly progressive and disabling, it is treatable. Appropriate management should minimise disability, improve breathlessness and reduce exacerbations*

## REFERENCES

Britton M (2003) The burden of COPD in the UK: results from the Confronting COPD survey. *Respiratory Medicine* 97(suppl C): S71–S79

Medical Research Council (1965) Definition and classification of chronic bronchitis for clinical and epidemiological purposes. *Lancet 1*, 775–779

National Collaborating Centre for Chronic Conditions (2004) Chronic obstructive pulmonary disease: National Clinical Guideline for management of chronic obstructive pulmonary disease in adults in primary and secondary care. *Thorax,* 59 (Suppl 1): 1–232. www.nice.org.uk/pdf/CG012_niceguideline.pdf

van Schayck CP, Loozen JMC, Wagena E, Akkermans RP, Wesseling GJ (2002) Detecting patients at high risk of developing chronic obstructive pulmonary disease in general practice: a cross sectional case finding study. *British Medical Journal* 324: 1370–1374

# PATIENT AND CARER INFORMATION:
## WHAT IS COPD?

- COPD is the term now used to describe chronic bronchitis and emphysema
- It causes progressive narrowing of the airways making it difficult to get air in and out of your lungs efficiently
- COPD also causes progressive destruction of the area of the lungs responsible for transferring oxygen from the air into the bloodstream and taking the waste gas, carbon dioxide, from the bloodstream to the air so that it can be breathed out
- Airway narrowing and disruption of gas exchange make you increasingly breathless during activity
- COPD is generally a direct result of cigarette smoking. Other factors such as exposure to dust and fumes at work may, occasionally, add to the effects of smoking but are rarely the only reason for the development of COPD
- The exception to this is a rare inherited problem called alpha 1 antitrypsin deficiency. This makes those affected extraordinarily susceptible to the harmful effects of cigarette smoke. There is usually a strong family history of COPD
- Stopping smoking is the only thing that will stop further damage to the lungs occurring. It is the most important thing that you can do, and is important no matter how bad the damage is
- COPD cannot be cured, but modern treatment is able to improve your symptoms, to keep you as active as possible for as long as possible, and will help to prevent bad attacks

## PRESENTATION

COPD generally presents after the age of 35 years. The symptoms include:

- Breathlessness on exertion
- Chronic cough
- Regular sputum production
- Frequent winter 'chest infections' or 'bronchitis'
- Wheeze

Many patients with COPD are not diagnosed until their disease is advanced because:

- Mild to moderate COPD may not cause any symptoms apart from a tendency to winter 'chest infections'
- The slowly progressive nature of the breathlessness allows patients to adapt unconsciously to progressive disability in the early stages of the disease
- The symptoms of chronic cough, sputum and breathlessness may be accepted as a normal consequence of smoking and their significance not appreciated
- Smokers with symptoms of COPD may be unwilling to seek medical help because they will 'only be told to stop smoking'

### VITAL POINTS

*COPD should be suspected in any patient over 35 years who is a current or former smoker and has one or more presenting symptoms*

*Pre-symptomatic COPD can be detected by performing screening spirometry on smokers over 35 years with a 'smokers' cough'*

## VITAL POINTS

* Early detection of COPD will allow effective targeting of smoking cessation support to this high risk group
* Smoking cessation at an early stage of the disease may prevent the development of severe, disabling COPD and thus be an extremely cost-effective intervention

## DIAGNOSIS 1: TAKING A HISTORY

### Current complaint

Allow the patient to give a short, uninterrupted history of their chest problems. A useful question is:

- 'Can we go right back to the beginning? When were you first aware of having any chest problems?'

You can then move on to elicit the following key points by direct questioning if necessary.

### Current symptoms

- 'When did you first notice breathing problems?'
  - Symptoms under the age of 35 years, or wheezing and 'chestiness' in childhood may indicate asthma
- 'Do you have good days and bad days?'
  - Asthma is characterised by variable symptoms
  - COPD is characterised by chronic, slowly progressive symptoms
- 'Do you cough and when is the cough worst?'
  - Waking at night with a cough is an important symptom of asthma and is unusual in mild to moderate COPD
  - Morning cough with clearance of sputum, after which the patient feels better, is common in COPD
  - Morning cough and chest tightness that continues for several hours is characteristic of asthma
- 'Do you bring up any phlegm/sputum when you cough?'
  - Morning sputum production is common in COPD

- Sputum production in asthma is variable and associated with exacerbations
- Production of large quantities of purulent sputum throughout the day is suggestive of bronchiectasis
- 'Do you get short of breath if you exert yourself?'
  - Ask if they are able to keep up with their peers when walking
  - Ask if they are able to walk and talk at the same time
- 'Have you noticed any wheezing or whistling noises in your chest?'
  - Wheeze is a feature of both asthma and COPD, but waking at night with wheeze is characteristic of asthma
  - Wheeze on exposure to allergens may indicate asthma

## Smoking history

- 'Have you ever been a smoker?'
  - A smoking history of 15–20 pack years, or more, is significant for COPD
  - Smoking pack years are used to assess an individual's total tobacco exposure: 20 cigarettes a day (a pack) for 1 year = 1 pack year. You will need to determine how many years they have smoked and how many they smoked a day (*see box*)

$$\frac{\text{No of cigarettes per day}}{20} \times \text{No of years smoked} = \text{Total pack years}$$

## Previous history of respiratory disease or atopic disease

- 'Have you ever been told you had asthma?' A previous history of asthma may indicate a recurrence of asthma
- 'Have you ever had eczema or hay fever?' Previous atopic disease makes late onset asthma more likely
- 'Did you have any serious chest infections in childhood?' Recurrent lower respiratory tract infection in childhood may suggest:
  - Previously undiagnosed asthma (this was often labelled 'bronchitis')
  - An additional risk factor for COPD
  - A cause of bronchiectasis

## Current and past medical history

- Co-morbidity is common in COPD and a history of other conditions should alert you to the possibility of other causes for the patient's symptoms. For example, shortness of breath can be due to either cardiac or respiratory disease, or both
- 'Do you have any other medical problems and have you had any serious medical problems or operations?'
  - Rheumatic fever can lead to heart valve damage and heart failure, which may present with similar symptoms to COPD
  - A combination of exertional breathlessness and 'chest tightness' may indicate angina
  - Think about malignant disease. Lung cancer can cause similar symptoms to COPD, as can secondary spread of cancer to the lungs from another organ such as the breast
  - Diabetes will increase the risk of ischaemic heart disease. This will need to be excluded as a cause of the patient's symptoms
- 'Do you suffer from high blood pressure or any heart problems?'
  - Cardiac causes for the patient's symptoms (particularly heart failure) will need to be excluded

## Family history

- 'Is there any family history of asthma or hay fever?'
  - A positive family history of atopic disease makes asthma more likely
- 'Is there any family history of COPD, or chronic bronchitis and emphysema?'
  - A positive family history of COPD increases the likelihood of COPD
  - A strong family history of COPD, particularly at a young age should raise the possibility of alpha 1 antitrypsin deficiency
- 'Is there a family history of heart disease?'
  - A positive family history of ischaemic heart disease will make cardiac causes for the patient's symptoms more likely

## Social history

- 'What occupations/jobs have you had?'
  - Exposure to dusts and fumes at work may increase the risk of developing COPD

- Coal miners may be eligible for compensation if they have COPD
- Exposure to known sensitising agents for occupational asthma may have given rise to persistent, severe occupational asthma. In this case the patient may be eligible for compensation
- 'What hobbies do you have?'
  - Keeping pigeons or other birds may cause 'pigeon fanciers' lung'
  - Wood working may give rise to occupational asthma

## Medication history

- 'What medicines do you take, both prescribed and bought over the counter at the chemist?'
  - The use of cardiac and anti-hypertensive medication will make cardiac causes for the patient's symptoms more likely
  - Beta-blocking medications (eg atenolol) can produce bronchospasm

### VITAL POINT

*✷ A thorough clinical history will help identify most cases of COPD and will ensure that other potential causes for the patient's symptoms are not overlooked*

## DIAGNOSIS 2: EXAMINATION

Clinical signs are usually absent in the early stages of COPD. In severe COPD the following clinical signs may be present:

- 'Barrel' (hyperinflated) chest:
  - Enlarged antero-posterior diameter of the thorax
  - Lowering of upper border of the liver on percussion – due to flattening of the diaphragm
  - Reduced distance between the cricoid bone and the top of the sternum
  - Widening of the angle between the lower rib and the xiphisternum
  - Paradoxical movement of the lower ribs
  - Reduced cardiac dullness on percussion due to hyperinflation of the lungs

- Accessory muscle use
- Wheeze, or quiet breath sounds on auscultation
- 'Purse-lip' breathing
- Peripheral oedema
- Central cyanosis
- Raised jugular venous pressure
- Excessive weight loss/cachexia

## VITAL POINT

* The presence of clinical signs is variable; they may be absent in some patients

### Spirometry

Measurement of lung function with a spirometer is essential for the early and accurate diagnosis of COPD:

- Spirometry can accurately identify airflow obstruction and differentiate obstructive and restrictive problems
- Measurement of peak expiratory flow (PEF) is insufficiently sensitive to detect airflow obstruction in mild COPD and may seriously underestimate the extent of obstruction in more severe disease
- Measurement of forced expiratory volume in one second ($FEV_1$) is necessary for staging the severity of airflow obstruction and as a guide to therapy
- $FEV_1$ is closely related to prognosis

## VITAL POINT

* Spirometry is essential for the diagnosis of COPD

### Lung function parameters

The essential lung function parameters to measure are:

- Slow vital capacity (VC, SVC or RVC) = the total volume of air exhaled in a relaxed manner from a position of maximum inhalation to maximum exhalation

- Forced vital capacity (FVC) = the total volume of air exhaled from a position of maximum inhalation to maximum exhalation using maximum effort
- Forced expiratory volume in one second ($FEV_1$) = the volume of air exhaled in the first second of an exhalation from maximum inhalation using maximum effort
- The ratio of $FEV_1$ to FVC ($FEV_1$%, or $FEV_1$/FVC) = the volume of air exhaled in the first second expressed as a percentage of the total volume of air exhaled from maximum inhalation to maximum exhalation. This is a marker of airflow obstruction

Predicted lung volumes are dependent on age, gender, height and ethnicity. The FVC and the $FEV_1$ are expressed as:

- An absolute value, in litres
- A percentage of the predicted value for a person of that age, gender, height and ethnic group
- In health:
  - The VC is the same as, or slightly less than the FVC
  - The FVC and $FEV_1$ are greater than 80% of their predicted value
  - The $FEV_1$% is greater than 70%

Respiratory and other conditions can affect the normal parameters of lung function.

- Conditions that obstruct airflow and produce obstructive spirometry include:
  - COPD
  - Asthma
- Conditions that reduce lung volumes but do not obstruct airflow produce restrictive spirometry. They include:
  - Diseases such as fibrosing alveolitis and pneumoconiosis that cause fibrosis of lung tissue
  - Pulmonary oedema
  - Gross obesity or skeletal deformity such as kyphoscoliosis
  - Previous surgery such as lobectomy or pneumonectomy
- Conditions that produce a mixed obstructive and restrictive pattern of spirometry include:
  - Severe airflow obstruction eg in advanced COPD
  - Severe bronchiectasis
  - Cystic fibrosis

|  | Normal spirometry | Obstruction | Restriction | Mixed obstruction and restriction |
|---|---|---|---|---|
| VC | Equal to or slightly less than FVC | Equal to or slightly greater than FVC | Equal to or slightly less than FVC | Usually greater then FVC |
| FVC | Over 80% predicted | Over 80% predicted | Less than 80% predicted | Less than 80% predicted |
| FEV$_1$ | Over 80% predicted | Less than 80% predicted | Less than 80% predicted | Less than 80% predicted |
| FEV$_1$ % | Over 70% (usually 75–80%) | Less than 70% | Over 75% (usually over 80–85%) | Less than 70% |

■ Volume/time trace:

♦ A spirometer should also produce a graph of volume exhaled against the time taken to exhale fully – the volume/time trace

♦ A normal volume/time trace has a typical shape

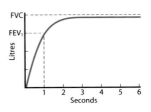

♦ An obstructive volume/time trace has a flattened shape

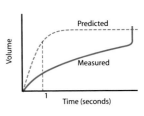

♦ A restrictive volume/time trace is a normal shape but smaller than normal

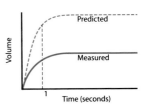

- In mixed obstruction and restriction the volume/time trace is flattened and small

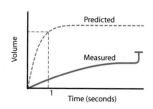

- The flow/volume trace:
  - Most modern electronic spirometers will also produce a graph of flow rate against volume – the flow volume trace

  - A normal flow/volume trace has a typical shape

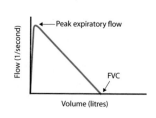

  - An obstructive flow/volume trace has a concave, 'scooped out' shape. This can be extremely useful for detecting very early airflow obstruction when the lung function parameters are still within normal limits and the volume/time trace looks normal

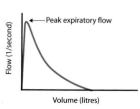

  - A restrictive flow/volume trace is narrow and domed

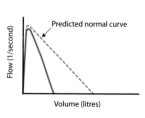

  - In severe COPD the flow/volume trace becomes scooped out and the FVC is reduced, giving a picture of mixed obstruction and restriction

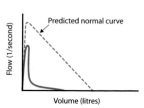

## EXCLUDING ALTERNATIVE DIAGNOSES

People susceptible to COPD are generally middle-aged or elderly smokers. They are also susceptible to other conditions that can be confused with COPD or will complicate its management.

### Asthma

Asthma and COPD can co-exist and cause similar symptoms. They can generally be differentiated by thorough history-taking.

|  | Asthma | COPD |
|---|---|---|
| Current or ex-smoker: 15–20+ pack years | Possibly | Nearly all |
| Symptoms under the age of 35 | Common | Uncommon |
| Chronic productive cough | Uncommon and variable | Common and persistent |
| Breathlessness | Variable day-to-day and diurnally | Persistent and progressive |
| Nocturnal waking with breathlessness or wheeze | Common | Uncommon |
| Family or personal history of atopy | Common | Uncommon |

If asthma is suspected or the diagnosis of COPD is in doubt, then consider

- Reversibility testing:
  - An increase of 400 ml or more in the $FEV_1$ following administration of a dose of bronchodilator (eg 200–400 µg salbutamol) suggests asthma
  - An increase of 400 µml or more in the $FEV_1$ following a 2-week course of 30 mg prednisolone daily suggests asthma
- Serial PEF:
  - Give the patient a PEF meter and ask them to record the highest of 3 readings in the morning and the evening over a 2-week period
  - Asthma is suggested if there is a 20% + variability *and* a minimum absolute change of more than 60 litres/minute on 3 days in a week over the 2-week period

## VITAL POINTS

*\* The role of reversibility testing is to differentiate asthma from COPD in those cases where the history is unclear. Reversibility testing cannot be used to identify which therapy is likely to be the most effective for long-term use*

*\* Reversibility testing and serial PEF should be carried out when the patient is clinically stable, not during an exacerbation*

## Chest X-ray

Routine chest X-ray should be carried out at the time of diagnosis:

- To exclude lung cancer (by the time the patient experiences symptoms most, although not all cancers will be visible on a chest X-ray)
- To detect enlargement of the heart and pulmonary oedema
- Hyperinflation of the lungs with flattening of the diaphragm will support a diagnosis of COPD, but may also be seen in chronic, severe asthma
- To detect large emphysematous bullae

## Cardiac causes of breathlessness

- Check the blood pressure
- If the patient is hypertensive and/or there is a previous history of cardiovascular disease consider electrocardiography and/or echocardiography

## Other investigations

- A full blood count should be taken in all patients at the time of diagnosis:
  - To exclude anaemia as a cause of breathlessness
  - To detect polycythaemia secondary to chronic hypoxia
- The body mass index (BMI) should be calculated as a baseline to enable early detection of weight loss
- Blood test for alpha 1 antitrypsin deficiency:
  - When patients present with COPD at a young age
  - When there is a strong family history of COPD
- Full pulmonary function tests, including gas transfer (TLCO) if:
  - Symptoms are disproportionate to the spirometry
  - There is doubt about the diagnosis
  - There is difficulty obtaining acceptable spirometry in the primary care setting
- Pulse oximetry should be considered:
  - If the patient is cyanosed or has ankle oedema
  - If the $FEV_1$ is less than 50% of the predicted value
- High resolution CT scanning is advisable if:
  - Bronchiectasis is suspected
  - Symptoms are disproportionate to the spirometry
  - There are abnormalities on the chest X-ray, such as emphysematous bullae
- Sputum culture should be considered if sputum is persistently purulent

---

### VITAL POINT

*✳ Alternative and co-morbid conditions must be considered as a cause of the patient's symptoms. If there is diagnostic doubt the patient should be referred for a specialist opinion*

# ASSESSING DISEASE SEVERITY

No single measurement can adequately assess the severity of COPD in an individual patient. Mild airflow obstruction can be associated with severe disability. Conversely, some patients with severe obstruction continue to function reasonably normally.

Assessment of severity of COPD should therefore encompass:

- Assessment of the severity of the airflow obstruction in terms of $FEV_1$:
    - Mild obstruction = $FEV_1$ 50–80% of predicted value
    - Moderate obstruction = $FEV_1$ 30–50% of predicted value
    - Severe obstruction = $FEV_1$ less than 30% of predicted value
- The frequency of exacerbations:
    - As COPD progresses, exacerbations tend to increase in frequency and severity
    - Frequent exacerbations are associated with accelerated loss of lung function and worsening health status
- Assessment of other factors known to affect prognosis:
    - BMI (weight loss is common in severe COPD and is associated with a poor prognosis; being overweight increases breathlessness and disability)
    - Breathlessness should be assessed using a validated scale such as the MRC dyspnoea scale (*see table*)

| The MRC Dyspnoea Scale |
|---|
| **1** Not troubled by breathlessness except on strenuous exercise |
| **2** Short of breath when hurrying on the level or walking up a slight hill |
| **3** Walks slower than people of the same age on the level because of breathlessness, or has to stop for breath when walking at own pace |
| **4** Stops for breath after walking about 100 metres or after a few minutes on the level |
| **5** Too breathless to leave the house or breathless when dressing or undressing |

- Exercise capacity (ask the patient how far they can walk and how much their breathlessness interferes with their ability to perform their daily tasks)

- Health status (ie an individual's perception of the impact of disease on their overall health condition and quality of life. Questions should cover the amount of fatigue experienced, emotional state and the extent to which they feel in control of their condition)
- The presence of cor pulmonale, as this is associated with severe disease and a poor prognosis. Warning signs include central cyanosis, peripheral oedema and raised JVP
- Measure oxygen saturation with a pulse oximeter if the $FEV_1$ is less than 50% of predicted value

## VITAL POINTS

\* *Assess dyspnoea regularly on the MRC scale. Offer pulmonary rehabilitation to those with a score of 3 or more*

\* *Depression and anxiety are common in severe COPD and respond well to conventional antidepressant and anxiolytic therapy*

\* *Refer for arterial blood gas estimation and assessment for long-term oxygen if the oxygen saturation is less than 92% at rest, breathing air, or there are other signs of cor pulmonale*

## REFERENCE

National Collaborating Centre for Chronic Conditions (2004) Chronic obstructive pulmonary disease: National Clinical Guideline for management of chronic obstructive pulmonary disease in adults in primary and secondary care. *Thorax* 59 (Suppl 1): 1–232

# 3 Stopping smoking

- Smoking is the major cause of COPD and smoking cessation the only thing that slows the relentless progression of the disease
- If a smoker is developing airflow obstruction, the sooner they stop smoking the better. However, it is never too late to stop!
- Cigarettes are the only legally sold product which, when used as intended, will kill 50% of its users
- Stopping smoking involves making considerable lifestyle changes
- Only 5–10% of quit attempts are successful, but the more attempts an individual makes the greater their chances of eventual success

## VITAL POINTS

*\* Nicotine is as addictive as cocaine or heroin and most addicted smokers will require help and support to stop*

*\* It usually takes several serious quit attempts before a smoker is able to quit completely*

## DEPENDENCE ON CIGARETTES

A heavily addicted smoker is likely to:

- Smoke the first cigarette of the day within 30 minutes of getting up
- Find it difficult to refrain from smoking in places where smoking is not allowed, such as in church, the theatre or at work
- Experience withdrawal symptoms when they are forced to go without cigarettes
- Smoke a pack or more of cigarettes a day and will inhale deeply, leaving a short 'stub'
- Want to smoke, even when they are too ill to get out of bed

The more heavily addicted the smoker the more likely they are to experience withdrawal symptoms and the more support they are likely to need.

## *Changing lifestyle*

Changing behaviour is acknowledged to be difficult. In order to change from being a smoker to a non-smoker, individuals need to:

- Perceive themselves to be at risk
- Believe that the risks are serious
- Believe that they are able to do something about stopping smoking
- Believe that the benefits of stopping smoking outweigh the costs (eg the discomforts of withdrawing from nicotine, the fear of being different from peers)

These beliefs can be a barrier to stopping smoking. For example:

- Smokers with a parent who smoked yet lived to a ripe old age may not perceive themselves to be at risk
- A smoker who 'just has a bit of a cough' may not perceive the risks to be serious
- They may not believe they are capable of stopping smoking eg if they have had several failed quit attempts in the past, or if they believe other factors in their lives, such as stress and family problems, make it impossible for them to stop
- They may feel that the problems associated with trying to stop smoking make it not worth the effort

Smokers may go through several stages before successfully stopping smoking:

- **Pre-contemplation (the contented smoker)** – they do not intend to stop smoking in the near future and they may not perceive smoking to be a problem
- **Contemplation** – they will consider stopping smoking but are not yet ready to do anything active about stopping
- **Preparation** – they are beginning to make plans to stop smoking and may already have started to make small changes, such as cutting down on the number they smoke, switching to lower tar cigarettes (neither strategy is likely to be successful on its own, but should be viewed as a step in the right direction)
- **Action** – they have stopped smoking, but are in the early (less than 6 months) stage of being a non-smoker
- **Maintenance** – they have managed not to smoke for 6 months or more

- **Relapse** – occasional lapses on the road to becoming a long-term quitter are normal and should be expected. However, relapse into regular smoking may also occur

## THE ROLE OF THE HEALTH PROFESSIONAL

In order to help smokers make the change from smoker to non-smoker you will need to be able to communicate effectively both verbally and non-verbally.

### Verbal communication

- Ask about smoking status in a non-confrontational way
- Use open, rather than closed questions to encourage discussion of the smoker's beliefs and attitudes to stopping smoking

| Open questions | Closed questions |
|---|---|
| How are you getting on with stopping smoking? | Have you given up smoking yet? |
| What do you think it would take to make you consider stopping smoking? | Don't you know that smoking is bad for you? |
| How do you feel about stopping smoking? | Wouldn't you like to stop smoking? |

- Closed questions provoke 'yes/no' answers and may antagonise smokers by 'putting them on the spot'
- Try to discover barriers to stopping smoking and help the smoker work out their own ways around them.

### Non-verbal communication

- Listen actively
- Make eye contact and look interested
- Nodding your head or making occasional non-verbal approving noises can be helpful – but don't overdo it

## Advising the 'contented' smoker

- Even brief intervention can trigger a smoker to think about quitting and begin to move through the stages of behaviour change
- Provide information about risk that is personalised, eg the effect of smoking in increasing the rate of lung function decline in COPD
- Help the smoker identify the benefits of quitting, eg stopping the rapid rate of lung function decline, reduction in cough and breathlessness etc
- Keep trying to motivate them to stop
- Record smoking status at every contact

## Advising smokers contemplating stopping

- Give clear, personalised advice to stop
- Ask if they are prepared to set a 'quit date' in the next month
- Help them to make a plan for stopping smoking
- Review previous quit attempts to discover previous reasons for failure
- Arrange a follow-up appointment

## Planning a quit attempt

- Discover how heavily addicted they are
- Encourage the use of nicotine replacement therapy or bupropion
- Set a date for stopping smoking completely
- Advise the smoker to tell their family and friends and try to elicit support from them. (Smokers who 'quit with a friend' are more likely to succeed)
- Keeping a smoking diary prior to the quit date may help identify potential danger times so that strategies for avoiding them can be formulated
- Help the smoker think about strategies for coping with challenges – eg other smokers (especially within the home), alcohol etc
- Advise the removal of all smoking materials on the night before quit day
- Advise that total abstinence is the best way to stop. Even a single cigarette can feed the addictive process and lead to failure

## Preventing relapse

- Arrange regular follow-up visits or phone calls
- Advise smokers about support services – eg Quitline – and encourage them to use them

- Give personalised advice about issues important to that smoker – eg weight gain, cravings, withdrawal symptoms
- Consider referring smokers who are unable to stop, despite repeated attempts and full support, to a specialist smoking cessation service

## The 'Five As'

- **ASK** – document smoking status at every visit
- **ADVISE** – urge smokers to quit
- **ASSESS** – willingness to quit. Ask if they are willing to set a quit date within the next 30 days
- **ASSIST** – with a quit plan, practical counselling, support and advice on the use of NRT or bupropion
- **ARRANGE** – follow-up contact, preferably on the quit day and within 2 weeks of quitting

### VITAL POINTS

\* *Helping your patients who smoke to stop is the most important thing you, as a health professional, can do to improve their health*

\* *Smokers who are followed up, advised and actively supported during a quit attempt are more likely to succeed. If resources are limited, concentrate support in the first 2 weeks of the attempt*

\* *It takes 3 months for the neurochemistry of a smoker to return to that of a non-smoker, and for the quit attempt to be considered truly successful*

## NICOTINE REPLACEMENT THERAPY (NRT)

- NRT aims to partially replace the nicotine from cigarettes:
  - It delivers a lower dose of nicotine at a slower rate and does not fuel nicotine addiction
  - It aims to provide a low, background level of nicotine to reduce cravings and withdrawal symptoms

- It should be used regularly for at least 8 weeks, after which the dose can be gradually reduced with the aim of stopping treatment completely after 12 weeks
- It is not suitable for genuinely light smokers
■ NRT is available as:
  - Transdermal patches – for 16 hour or 24 hour use
  - Chewing gum
  - Lozenges
  - Sub-lingual tablets
  - Inhalator
  - Nasal spray
■ All forms of NRT are effective and the choice of formulation is a matter of the smoker's personal preference
■ All forms of NRT are available on prescription or over the counter at pharmacies

## Contraindications and side effects of NRT

■ Contraindications include:
  - Recent (within 3 months) heart attack or stroke
  - Active peptic ulceration
  - Pregnancy
  - Breastfeeding
■ Continuing to smoke while using NRT is potentially dangerous and the quit attempt is likely to fail
■ Side effects include:
  - Local irritation (with patches)
  - Sleep disturbance or insomnia
■ The side effects of NRT are the same as those associated with smoking. As a general rule the benefits of using NRT to help a smoker quit far outweigh the risks of continued smoking

## BUPROPION

- Bupropion (Zyban™) works directly on the addiction pathways of the brain and prevents 'cravings', rather than replacing one nicotine delivery system with another
- Bupropion is only available on prescription
- One 150 mg tablet is taken daily for 6 days; then one 150 mg tablet twice daily (at least 8 hours apart) for the remainder of the 2 month course of treatment
- A 'quit date' is set 10–17 days into the course of treatment
- Treatment is continued for 2 months, but if the smoker has been unable to stop smoking completely by the end of the first month then consideration should be given to stopping treatment as the quit attempt is unlikely to be successful
- Bupropion is not suitable for the smoker who is not committed to stopping

### Contraindications and side effects of bupropion

- Bupropion is generally well tolerated, but prescribers need to be aware of some important contraindications:
  - Current or past seizure
  - Use of medications that lower the seizure threshold, eg antidepressants, antipsychotics or theophyllines
  - Current or past eating disorder, eg anorexia or bulimia
  - History of bipolar disorder, eg manic depressive psychosis
  - Hepatic cirrhosis
  - Brain tumour or previous severe head injury
  - Withdrawal from alcohol or benzodiazepines

- Side effects of bupropion include:
  - Insomnia
  - Dry mouth
  - Generalized rash
  - Nausea
  - Agitation
- There have been some highly publicised deaths associated with bupropion. However, a causal link between bupropion use and these deaths is disputed
- The risks of continuing to smoke far outweigh the risk of using bupropion, provided it is prescribed with care to appropriate people

## VITAL POINTS

\* *Consult the British National Formulary for a full list of contraindications and cautions and take a full medical and drug history (including the use of over-the-counter medications) before prescribing bupropion*

\* *Nicotine replacement therapy or bupropion can double the chances of quitting*

## REFERENCES

NICE (2002) Guidance on the use of nicotine replacement therapy (NRT) and bupropion for smoking cessation. *Technology appraisal guidance* No 38.
www.nice.org.uk/article.asp?a=30631
Raw M, McNeill A, West R (1998) Smoking cessation guidelines for health professionals. *Thorax* 53(Suppl 5): S1–S38
www.brit-thoracic.org.uk/public_content.asp?pageid+7&catid_368&subcatid+158
West R, McNeill A, Raw M (2000) Smoking cessation guidelines for health professionals: an update. *Thorax* 55: 987–999
www.brit-thoracic.org.uk/public_content.asp?pageid+7&catid_368&subcatid+158

- Stopping smoking is the single, most important thing you can do to help yourself

- Stopping smoking is something you need to plan. Set a quit date – preferably within the next month and begin to prepare to become an ex-smoker

- Keep a smoking diary for a couple of weeks. Record the time of day and the circumstances when you smoke and note whether you really wanted that cigarette. It will help you recognise which are the most difficult cigarettes of the day to give up, so that you can plan ways of avoiding those 'danger' times

- Think of an activity to help you avoid the danger times. For example, if you always smoke with a cup of coffee, try having a glass of water. If you smoke after a meal, get up and wash up straight away, or go for a walk instead

- If possible try to stop smoking with a friend or another family member. You can support each other and are more likely to be successful

- Tell your family and friends that you are stopping smoking so that they don't inadvertently put temptation in your way. If they deliberately try to make you start smoking again they are not your friends. Avoid them for the first few weeks!

- Use the support offered by your nurse or doctor. They will be glad to help you

- The smoking cessation 'Quit' helpline can be useful. Make a note of the number and call it if you are having difficulties

- Cutting down gradually or changing to a low tar brand is not effective in helping you to stop. You should aim to stop smoking completely on 'quit day'

- The night before your chosen quit day, get rid of all your smoking materials (cigarettes, ash trays, lighters etc). This will remove temptation during the critical early days

- Consider using nicotine replacement or the anti-smoking tablet, Zyban. They have been extensively tested and will double your chances of stopping smoking for good. Your doctor, nurse or pharmacist will be able to help you chose the best form of treatment for you
- Use nicotine replacement therapy for the full course and don't be tempted to cut down on its use too early. Failure is usually due to not using it regularly enough in the early stages, or stopping using it too soon
- When you stop smoking put aside the money you would have spent on cigarettes. You will be surprised how quickly it will build up. After a week or fortnight, spend the money on a treat for yourself as a reward for not smoking
- Stopping smoking may make you hungry, especially for sweet things. It is better to keep a 'nibble box' of non-fattening foods such as raw carrot or celery
- Weight gain is usual. Most people will put on about 8 lbs. This weight gain is far less of a health hazard than smoking and fear of gaining weight should not be a barrier to you stopping smoking
- Don't try to diet and stop smoking at the same time. Avoid sucking sweets or eating fattening foods and, as you begin to feel fitter, start taking exercise. This can help distract you from cravings and will help your general fitness and reduce your weight gain
- Cravings are short lived. Plan ways to distract yourself and they will pass quickly. The longer you stay off cigarettes the fewer cravings you will experience
- Avoid going to the pub for the first couple of weeks. Alcohol will reduce your willpower
- Take it one day at a time. Tell yourself, 'Today, I am not going to have a cigarette'
- If you don't succeed this time – work out what went wrong, make plans to avoid that situation next time and TRY AGAIN!

# 4  How to manage COPD – drug therapy

Asthma patients who have developed a degree of fixed airflow obstruction should be treated along asthma management guidelines. They will continue to need inhaled corticosteroids and will probably need to be treated according to Step 3 or 4 of the BTS/SIGN guidelines.

The aims of management of COPD are to:

- Reduce breathlessness and exercise limitation
- Reduce the frequency of exacerbations
- Reduce symptoms of chronic cough
- Treat anxiety and depression

## BRONCHODILATORS

- Bronchodilators are the mainstay of therapy for COPD. They can:
  - Reduce breathlessness
  - Improve exercise tolerance
  - Increase feelings of wellbeing
- Bronchodilators may not produce significant improvements in the $FEV_1$, but appear to work by reducing both static and dynamic hyperinflation of the lungs. This is the probable explanation for their clinical effectiveness
- The efficacy of treatment should not be assessed in terms of improvements in lung function alone. Subjective assessment of symptomatic improvement is a relevant and effective way of assessing therapeutic response
- The following 5 questions are a quick and effective method of assessing response to treatment:
  - 'Has your treatment made a difference to you?'
  - 'Is your breathing easier in any way?'
  - 'Can you do some things now that you couldn't do before, or the same things but faster?'

- 'Can you do the same things as before, but are now less breathless when you do them?'
- 'Has your sleep improved?'

## VITAL POINTS

*※ Individual response to different classes of bronchodilator varies between patients. Different drugs and combinations should be trialled for several weeks and responses assessed in terms of subjective symptomatic improvement*

*※ Complicated medication regimens with multiple drugs are a significant problem for COPD patients. Every effort should be made to simplify treatment regimens*

## Short-acting bronchodilators

### Short-acting beta2 agonists

- Beta2 agonist bronchodilators have a rapid onset of action and are therefore suitable for use on an 'as needed' basis for immediate symptom relief at all stages of COPD severity, as well as regularly as background treatment
- 'As needed' short-acting beta2 agonists may be the only therapy required for patients with mild COPD who are only occasionally troubled by breathlessness, or are breathless during exacerbations only
- Stimulation of beta receptors in areas other than airway smooth muscle, such as the heart and skeletal muscle, may give rise to side effects of palpitations, cardiac arrhythmia and tremor
- In practice, side effects are rare with standard doses and, when they occur, tend to be transient and disappear with continued usage
- Cardiovascular side effects may be relevant with high doses, such as those given via nebuliser, in elderly patients with co-morbid cardiovascular disease. Caution should be exercised
- High doses of short-acting beta2 agonists may reduce serum potassium levels. This may be particularly important for elderly patients who tend to tolerate biochemical disturbance poorly, and may also be taking diuretics (which reduce potassium levels)

Short-acting beta2 agonists are available in the following forms:

- Salbutamol is available in a pressurised metered dose inhaler (pMDI), in a breath activated pMDI, in a variety of dry powder inhalers (DPI) and as a nebuliser solution
- The standard dose of salbutamol is 200–400 µgm 4–6 hourly or as needed
- The standard dose via a nebuliser is 2.5–5 mg 4–6 hourly
- Terbutaline is available as a DPI in the Turbohaler. It is also available as a nebuliser solution
- The standard dose of terbutaline is 500 µgm 4–6 hourly or as needed
- The standard dose of terbutaline via nebuliser is 5–10 mg 4–6 hourly

## VITAL POINT

*✻ Patients taking regular, nebulised short-acting beta2 agonists should have their serum potassium checked every 6 months, particularly if they are also taking diuretics and/or theophylline*

### Short-acting anticholinergics

- Increased resting muscle tone in airway smooth muscle (bronchomotor tone) is an important component of airflow obstruction in COPD
- Anticholinergic bronchodilators block the action of acetylcholine, the neurotransmitter of the parasympathetic nervous system, and reduce resting bronchomotor tone
- Anticholinergic bronchodilators may be of particular benefit in COPD
- Anticholinergics have a longer onset of action than short-acting beta2 agonists making them less suitable for immediate symptom relief. They are generally used regularly 3–4 times daily
- They are poorly systemically absorbed and therefore cause few side effects
- The commonest side effect is a dry mouth. Although they could, theoretically lead to problems with accommodation, constipation and urinary retention, in practice they are generally safe and well-tolerated

Ipratropium bromide is available as a pMDI, as a DPI in capsules for use through the Aerohaler and as a nebuliser solution:

- The standard dose via pMDI is 40–80 μgm 6–8 hourly
- The standard dose via Aerohaler is 40 μgm 6–8 hourly
- The standard dose via nebuliser is 250–500 μgm 6–8 hourly

### Combination therapy

- A combination of short-acting beta2 agonist and anticholinergic may provide better symptom relief for some patients
- The use of a combination inhaler may simplify treatment regimen
- Combination therapy should be tried if patients remain symptomatic on monotherapy of short-acting bronchodilators

A combination of salbutamol and ipratropium is available as Combivent® in pMDI and nebuliser solution:

- The standard dose of drug via pMDI is 2–4 puffs 3–4 times daily. This will give 200–400 μgm of salbutamol and 40–80 μgm ipratropium 3–4 times daily
- A 'nebule' of Combivent via a nebuliser delivers 2.5 mg salbutamol and 500 μgm of ipratropium bromide. It is generally given 3–4 times daily
- A combination of fenoterol and ipratropium is available as Duovent® nebuliser solution. A 'nebule' of Duovent delivers 1.25 mg of fenoterol and 500 μgm of ipratropium bromide

### Long-acting bronchodilators

- Patients whose symptoms are not optimally controlled by regular short-acting bronchodilators and/or combinations of short-acting beta2 agonists and short-acting anticholinergics should be given long-acting bronchodilators
- Long-acting bronchodilators should also be considered if patients have 2 or more exacerbations a year as they may help to reduce frequency of exacerbations

## Long-acting beta2 agonists

- Long-acting beta2 agonists have a duration of action of 12 hours, making them suitable for twice daily use
- Long-acting beta2 agonists have similar bronchodilator effects to short-acting agents, but appear to also have some additional benefits:
  - Improved health-related quality of life
  - Reduced exacerbation frequency
- The side effects of long-acting beta2 agonists are similar to the short-acting agents

Clinical trials have shown that salmeterol and formoterol have similar clinical effects:

- Both salmeterol and formoterol are licensed for use in COPD without concomitant inhaled corticosteroid
- Salmeterol is available as pMDI and as a DPI via Accuhaler or Diskhaler
- The dose of salmeterol is 50 µgm twice daily. No benefit is gained from higher doses and the incidence of side effects is increased
- Formoterol is available as a DPI via Turbohaler or DPI capsule via the Aeroliser
- The dose of formoterol is 12 µgm twice daily

## Long-acting anticholinergics

- Tiotropium bromide is the only available long-acting anticholinergic. It has a duration of action of 24 hours, making it suitable for once-daily use
- It appears to have better bronchodilator effects than ipratropium and similar additional benefits to long-acting beta2 agonists
- Tiotropium bromide is currently only available as a DPI capsule for use through the Handihaler. The dose of tiotropium is 18 µgm once daily

## Oral beta2 agonist bronchodilators

- Whenever possible inhaled bronchodilators should be used as they have a more rapid onset of action and are less likely to cause side effects
- Oral beta2 agonists should be reserved for those few patients who are unable or unwilling to use inhalers
- Availability is as follows:
  - Slow release salbutamol tablets, 8 mg twice daily
  - Bambuterol (a precursor of terbutaline), 10–20 mgs at night

## Theophyllines

- Theophyllines have been used to treat airflow obstruction for around 100 years
- The therapeutic range for theophyllines is narrow (10–20 mg/litre). They are potentially toxic and interact with a large number of other drugs. Side effects are often troublesome and some are life-threatening
- Difficulties with theophylline use has largely consigned them to second or third line therapy
- They should only be used after adequate trials of short-acting and long-acting bronchodilators, or if patients are unable to use inhaled therapy

## INHALER DEVICES

- Hand-held inhaler devices (including a spacer if appropriate) are the preferred method of delivering inhaled therapy
- The choice of inhaler device should depend on the patient's ability to use the inhaler and on their preference
- Ideally, the device should be portable, discreet and easy to use
- Spacers should be compatible with the pMDI and should be used by putting one puff at a time into the spacer, followed by a single, slow, deep inhalation or several tidal breaths

- Spacers should be washed in water and washing-up liquid and left to air dry not more than once a month
- Regular nebulised bronchodilators should only be considered for patients with severe and distressing breathlessness despite optimal bronchodilator therapy with a hand-held inhaler
- Patients being considered for long-term nebulised therapy should be seen by a specialist experienced in nebuliser use who will:
  - Assess the patient's need for therapy and their response to it
  - Supply and maintain the equipment, and educate patients and carers in its use
  - Provide long-term support and supervision
- Nebuliser therapy should only be continued if it has been shown to produce one or more of the following:
  - A reduction in symptoms
  - An improvement in exercise capacity
  - Improved ability to perform normal activities of daily living
  - An improvement in lung function
- Drugs for use with a nebuliser are expensive; nebulised therapy can be restrictive and time-consuming for patients
- Nebuliser equipment is not available on prescription. It is inappropriate to suggest that patients purchase their own
- A general practice that loans nebuliser equipment to a patient is responsible for ensuring that it has an electrical safety check every year and is appropriately maintained and serviced
- The ability of patients and their carers to use and care for nebuliser equipment should be carefully checked

## VITAL POINTS

* Inhaler technique should be taught and regularly checked by a health professional who is familiar with inhalers and competent in their use
* If domiciliary nebulised therapy is prescribed, the patient should be provided with the equipment and a regular supply of disposables, servicing, advice and support

## CORTICOSTEROIDS

### *Inhaled corticosteroids (IHCS)*

- None of the currently available IHCS are licensed on their own for use in COPD

- IHCS do not significantly reduce lung function decline or affect the natural history of COPD at any stage of the disease, and they are of no benefit to patients with mild COPD ($FEV_1$ greater than 50% of predicted value)

- Patients with more severe COPD ($FEV_1$ less than 50% of predicted value) may benefit from long-term IHCS in terms of reduced exacerbation rates and a reduced health status decline

- NICE recommends IHCS be considered for patients with an $FEV_1$ equal to or less than 50% predicted value, who have also had 2 or more exacerbations requiring antibiotics or oral corticosteroids in the previous 12 months

- Oral corticosteroid trials cannot be used to predict which patients will benefit from long-term IHCS

- The optimum IHCS compound and the optimum dose is not yet known although meta analysis suggests that moderate to high doses (1000 µgm of beclometasone or its equivalent /day) are effective and lower doses are not

- There are several studies of the effects of IHCS in COPD patients over 3 years, but the longer term effects of high dose IHCS on, for example, bone density have not yet been determined

- High dose IHCS are associated with local side effects – oral thrush and hoarse voice. The use of a large volume spacer can reduce these side effects and patients should be advised to rinse their mouth, gargle and spit after using their IHCS inhaler

- Consideration should be given to the risk of osteoporosis, cataracts and other side effects in patients treated with high dose IHCS. These risks should be discussed with patients

### Combined IHCS and long-acting beta2 agonist (LABA) inhalers

- Combination inhalers of IHCS and LABA provide:
  - Better improvement in lung function when compared to both separate components and placebo
  - Improvement in quality of life
  - Reduced frequency of exacerbations
- Combination inhalers may be more convenient for patients
- They should be considered for patients:
  - With an $FEV_1$ equal to or less than 50% predicted value
  - Who are experiencing 2 or more exacerbations a year
  - Who have shown good symptomatic response to a LABA
- Availability is as follows:
  - A combination of formoterol 12 µgm and budesonide 400 µgm twice daily as the DPI Symbicort Turbohaler
  - A combination of salmeterol 50 µgm and fluticasone 500 µgm twice daily as the DPI Seretide 500 Accuhaler

### Oral corticosteroids

- Oral corticosteroids are used in short courses (30 mg prednisolone daily for up to 2 weeks) to treat exacerbations of COPD

- Maintenance oral corticosteroids should not normally be used as they are associated with significant and potentially serious side effects
- However, some patients with very severe COPD deteriorate when a short course of oral corticosteroids is withdrawn following an exacerbation. Such patients may require maintenance oral steroids
- Patients under the age of 65 who require maintenance oral corticosteroids should be monitored for osteoporosis and given appropriate prophylaxis
- Patients over the age of 65 on maintenance oral corticosteroids should be started on osteoporosis prophylaxis without the need for monitoring
- Patients on maintenance oral corticosteroids or requiring frequent short courses should be considered for specialist assessment and supervision

## VITAL POINT

*\* The dose of maintenance oral corticosteroids should be kept as low as possible*

## OTHER DRUGS

### Mucolytics

- Mucolytics increase expectoration of sputum by reducing its viscosity
- They can reduce the number of exacerbations and improve symptoms of cough and sputum production
- They should be considered for patients with chronic cough and sputum and continued if they improve symptoms
- Availability is as follows:
  - Carbocisteine 750 mg three times daily, reducing to 1.5 gm daily in divided doses
  - Mecysteine 200 mg 4 times daily for 2 days, then 200 mg thrice daily for 6 weeks, reducing to 200 mg twice daily

### Anxiolytics and antidepressants

- COPD produces disabling and distressing symptoms which can lead to social isolation, anxiety and depression

- The symptoms and signs of depression can be similar to those of COPD and are often overlooked
- Patients with severe COPD are 2.5 times more likely to be depressed than healthy individuals. Patients who are hypoxic or severely breathless are at particular risk
- Depression and anxiety worsen quality of life and increase the psychosocial problems associated with COPD
- Depressed COPD patients are more likely to be admitted to hospital
- Conventional anxiolytic and antidepressant drugs are effective for COPD patients

## VITAL POINT

* *The benefits of treating anxiety and depression alongside COPD need to be fully discussed with patients in order for treatment to be accepted*

## REFERENCES

British Thoracic Society (1997) Current best practice for nebuliser treatment. *Thorax* 52 (Suppl 2). www.brit-thoracic.org.uk/public_content.asp

British Thoracic Society, Scottish Intercollegiate Guidelines Network (2004). *British guideline on the management of asthma.* www.brit-thoracic.org.uk/docs/asthmafull.pdf

Burge PS, Calverley PMA, Jones PW et al (2000) Randomised, double blind, placebo controlled study of fluticasone propionate in patients with moderate to severe chronic obstructive pulmonary disease: the ISOLDE trial. *British Medical Journal* 320: 1297–1303

Jones PW, Bellamy D, Crockett AWB et al (2001) *Assessing treatment outcomes in COPD.* London: Synergy Medical Education

National Collaborating Centre for Chronic Conditions (2004). Chronic obstructive pulmonary disease: National Clinical Guideline for management of chronic obstructive pulmonary disease in adults in primary and secondary care. *Thorax* 59 (Suppl 1), 1–232. www.nice.org.uk/pdf/CG012_niceguideline.pdf

Shah P, Dhurjon L, Metcalfe T, Gibson JM (1992) Acute angle closure glaucoma associated with nebulised ipratropium bromide and salbutamol. *British Medical Journal* 304, 40–41

# PATIENT AND CARER INFORMATION

## MEDICATIONS USED TO TREAT COPD

- The aim of treatment for COPD is to reduce symptoms and attacks and to enable you to keep as active as possible

- Inhalers are the best way of getting treatment into the lungs where they are needed. Inhaled medication works quicker, is more effective and causes fewer side effects than tablets

- You should be shown how to use your inhaler and your doctor or nurse will need to check regularly how you are using it

- The inhalers are safe and not addictive. You will not become dependent on them and there is no benefit in trying to do without them

- Bronchodilators work by opening the airways and reducing the amount of air trapped in the lungs, making it easier and more comfortable to breathe

- Taking a dose of quick acting bronchodilator (usually a blue inhaler) before doing something that you know will make you breathless can help prevent or reduce the problem. Your doctor or nurse will be able to tell you which one of your inhalers you should take

- Carry a blue, bronchodilator inhaler with you when you leave your home to relieve attacks of breathlessness quickly, if they occur

- If you are prescribed long-acting bronchodilator treatments, you should take them regularly, as prescribed

- Theophylline tablets are occasionally used to treat COPD. However, they can have unpleasant side effects, which should be explained to anyone taking them

- Inhalers containing steroids are sometimes used to help prevent severe attacks. Inhalers deliver the drug directly to the lungs where it is needed and do not cause serious side effects

- Steroid inhalers need to be taken regularly, as prescribed, if they are to be effective

- Steroid inhalers sometimes cause minor, local problems in the mouth and throat. They can make you more prone to fungal infections and they may make your voice hoarse. These problems can generally be avoided by making sure that you rinse your mouth out, gargle and spit after using the inhaler

- Taking the inhaler through a large plastic spacer, which can be left at home and does not need to be carried about, also reduces these problems

- Two-week courses of steroid tablets are sometimes used to treat bad attacks of COPD. Used in this way they will not cause serious side effects. Some people feel a little euphoric or hungry when they are taking them

- Steroid tablets can occasionally cause indigestion. This needs to be reported to the doctor who will advise you whether to continue

- Some steroid tablets should be taken before food and others after. The doctor, nurse or pharmacist should tell you how to take the ones you have been prescribed

- A few people with very severe COPD need to take steroid tablets every day over long periods

- If you have been prescribed steroid tables for more than 3 weeks it is very important not to stop taking them abruptly. Your doctor or nurse will give you instructions about how to reduce the dose gradually to allow your body time to adjust

- COPD can cause anxiety and depression which, in turn will worsen symptoms and reduce your ability to cope. There is effective treatment available for anxiety and depression, which will improve your quality of life and ability to cope with the symptoms of COPD

# 5 Pulmonary rehabilitation

*'Pulmonary rehabilitation is a multi-disciplinary programme of care for patients with chronic respiratory impairment that is individually tailored and designed to optimise physical and social performance and autonomy'* (NICE 2004)

- Progressive breathlessness on exertion leads to exercise avoidance and reduced levels of activity; lack of activity leads to loss of fitness and increasing breathlessness on exertion
- Reduced functional ability can lead to social isolation, loss of self-esteem, anxiety and depression
- Pulmonary rehabilitation aims to break the cycle of increasing inactivity and loss of fitness. It also aims to increase COPD patients' understanding of their disease and their ability and confidence to manage themselves

## BENEFITS

Pulmonary rehabilitation is extremely effective and can produce significant and meaningful improvements in functional ability and quality of life for COPD patients. The British Thoracic Society has identified the benefits as:

- Significant improvements in functional ability
- Greater maximum exercise capacity
- Improved quality of life
- Reduced breathlessness
- Reduced number of hospital admissions
- Reduced health service utilisation

## VITAL POINT

*✳ There is good evidence that pulmonary rehabilitation is cost effective and the benefits last at least 2 years*

# COMPONENTS OF THE PROGRAMME

Programmes should last a minimum of 6 weeks with at least 2 supervised group sessions a week.

## Exercise

The core component of pulmonary rehabilitation is individually prescribed physical exercise:

- Aerobic exercise to increase cardiovascular fitness
  - Peripheral muscle strengthening
  - Some centres also include respiratory muscle exercises
- Exercise is undertaken 3 times a week, including at least 2 supervised sessions
- Patients are expected to continue to exercise at home and may be asked to keep an exercise diary
- The intensity of the exercise is prescribed according to the patient's baseline exercise capacity (determined using validated and standardised tests such as the 6-minute walk test or incremental shuttle walk test)
- Exercise is geared to improving functional ability and endurance, and includes walking or cycling for a minimum of 20–30 minutes
- Exercise intensity is increased throughout the programme as the patient's fitness improves
- Peripheral muscle strengthening exercises improve functional ability. Upper limb exercises are particularly helpful
- Rehabilitation aims to change behaviour so that patients continue to exercise after completing the programme

## Education

- Education, although an important part of a pulmonary rehabilitation programme, is not effective on its own for improving quality of life and exercise capacity
- The educational component of a programme can be adapted to suit the needs of an individual group. Suggested topics include:
  - The lungs in health and disease
  - Medication – including inhaler techniques and oxygen therapy
  - Managing symptoms

- ◆ Making lifestyle changes (eg stopping smoking)
- ◆ Physical exercise and its benefits
- ◆ Relaxation and energy conservation
- ◆ Managing exacerbations and self-management plans
- ◆ Diet and nutrition
- ◆ Travel and making the most of life with COPD
- ◆ Benefits and how to obtain them
- ◆ Support networks
- ◆ End of life decision making and advanced directives
- Most programmes actively encourage relatives and carers to attend
- Effective education sessions encourage interaction from patients and their relatives, are relevant and specific and put the patient in control

## Psychosocial support

- Pulmonary rehabilitation is most effective when carried out in a group setting, as patients benefit from peer support and encouragement
- Many programmes 'graduate' patients to a patient support group, such as Breathe Easy, where they can continue to benefit from peer support

## THE MULTI-DISCIPLINARY TEAM

Key members of the pulmonary rehabilitation team include:

- Physiotherapists
- Specialist nurses
- Doctors

Other team members are recruited according to local need and availability. They include:

- Pharmacists
- Occupational therapists
- Dietitians
- Clinical psychologists
- Social workers
- Patient support group representatives (see page 109)

# SELECTING PATIENTS FOR REHABILITATION

NICE recommends pulmonary rehabilitation be offered to all COPD patients who are disabled by their disease (ie to all patients who have to walk more slowly than their peers because of breathlessness, or have to stop to get their breath when walking at their own pace).

- Pulmonary rehabilitation is appropriate for all patients who are aware of being disabled by their symptoms and at all stages of the disease
- Patients should be referred when they are clinically stable and when medical management has been optimised
- Patients with severe co-morbidity that limits ability to exercise – eg unstable angina or severe arthritis – may not be able to exercise fully. They can still benefit from the educational aspects and peer support but are unlikely to gain as much
- Patients who are committed to undertaking a programme but are current smokers should not be excluded. Improving their self-esteem and function and giving them access to a peer group who have successfully stopped smoking may be beneficial
- Oxygen dependency is not a barrier. Such patients can still benefit
- Patients who continue to work may find attendance difficult
- Patients from ethnic minority groups may experience language difficulties. Translation services may be needed. Where there is a large ethnic minority a separate programme for this group may be an option
- Transport may be problematic if the patient has to travel a distance to the rehabilitation centre
- Patients who are very elderly, or are hypoxic may have impaired learning abilities. Special consideration may also need to be given to patients with visual or hearing difficulties
- Patients need to be fully informed about the potential benefits of rehabilitation and the commitment they need to give to gain benefit
- Misconceptions about rehabilitation need to be explored

## VITAL POINT

❋ *No patient is too sick or too well to benefit from pulmonary rehabilitation*

## SERVICE PROVISION

- Programmes should be available to all suitable patients, in locations that are convenient and accessible, within a reasonable period of referral

- Pulmonary rehabilitation is 'low tech' and does not require expensive exercise equipment. It can be delivered effectively in church halls (for example), provided appropriate, trained personnel are available

- Most UK programmes are currently run in secondary care settings, although community based programmes are becoming more common

- Despite ample evidence for its effectiveness, current service provision is poor

## VITAL POINT

*❋ Patients, their doctors, nurses and physiotherapists should lobby their primary care trusts for better provision of pulmonary rehabilitation services*

## REFERENCES

British Lung Foundation, British Thoracic Society (2003) *Pulmonary Rehabilitation Survey*. London: British Lung Foundation. www.brit-thoracic.org.uk/docs/PulRehamJUN03.pdf

British Thoracic Society (2001) Pulmonary rehabilitation. *Thorax*, 56(11): 827–834. www.brit-thoracic.org.uk/docs/Pulmonaryrehab.pdf

Calverley P, Bellamy D (2000) The challenge of providing better care for patients with chronic obstructive pulmonary disease. *Thorax*, 55: 78–82

Menier RJ (1994) Benefits of a multidisciplinary pulmonary rehabilitation program (letter). *Chest*, 105: 640–641

National Collaborating Centre for Chronic Conditions (2004) Chronic obstructive pulmonary disease: National Clinical Guideline for management of chronic obstructive pulmonary disease in adults in primary and secondary care. *Thorax*, 59 (Suppl 1): 1–232. www.nice.org.uk/pdf/CG012_niceguideline.pdf

# PATIENT AND CARER INFORMATION

- Pulmonary rehabilitation is an exercise and education programme for people with chronic lung problems. Its aims are to reduce breathlessness, enable you to do more and improve quality of life

- Before starting the programme you will be assessed by a physiotherapist, who will find out what you are able to do and prescribe an individual exercise programme based on this assessment

- During your assessment you will be asked to complete some questionnaires that will help identify your particular problems. These can then be addressed during the programme, so that you get the best possible benefit

- The exercise you are prescribed is designed to make you moderately short of breath. Regular exercise at this level will improve your fitness and help to reduce your breathlessness. It will not do you any harm

- You will not be expected to do anything that makes you distressingly short of breath. Trained physiotherapists and nurses will supervise your exercise and ensure your safety and comfort

- You do not need any special shoes or clothing. Loose, comfortable clothes and flat shoes are all that is needed

- During and after the rehabilitation programme you will be expected to commit to undertaking some regular gentle exercise, usually walking. By exercising regularly, you will gain most (and most lasting) benefit from the programme

- Exercise sessions form only part of a rehabilitation programme. Time is also set aside for various professionals to come and talk about COPD and how you can best look after yourself. This is your opportunity to ask questions and air any concerns you have

- Your relatives or carers will be invited to attend sessions with you. This gives them the opportunity to discuss their concerns too

- Pulmonary rehabilitation is undertaken in a group. Group members will have similar problems and can usually help and support each other

- Pulmonary rehabilitation has been widely researched. It is safe and effective. Most people who undertake a programme find it beneficial

# 6   Oxygen therapy

Oxygen can improve exercise capacity and improve survival in patients with chronic hypoxia but, until recently, it was often prescribed haphazardly.

## LONG-TERM OXYGEN THERAPY (LTOT)

- LTOT, when used for 15 hours a day or more, has been shown to improve survival in patients with chronic hypoxia
- Without LTOT the prognosis of these patients is poor. Nearly 60% will die within 3 years
- Other benefits of LTOT in chronically hypoxic COPD patients include:
  - Improved exercise tolerance
  - Improved appetite and general well-being
  - Reduced ankle oedema
  - Reduced hospital admissions

### Identifying patients for assessment for LTOT

- Consider the need for LTOT in all patients with:
  - An $FEV_1$ less than 30% predicted value
  - Cyanosis
  - Polycythaemia
  - Peripheral oedema
  - Raised jugular venous pressure
  - Pulse oximetry readings of 92% *or less*
- Patients with less severe COPD ($FEV_1$ 30–49% predicted) may also benefit if they have any of the above features of chronic hypoxia and cor pulmonale
- Measure oxygen saturation with a pulse oximeter in all patients with an $FEV_1$ of less than 50% predicted as a routine. This will ensure that all patients who might benefit from LTOT are identified at an early stage

## Patient assessment

- Patients should be assessed during a stable period, at least 4 weeks after an exacerbation, and should be on optimal medical management

- Arterial blood gases should be assessed on 2 occasions, at least 3 weeks apart

- The current criteria for LTOT are:
  - $PaO_2$ less than 7.3 kPa, or
  - $PaO_2$ between 7.3 and 8 kPa and one or more of:
  - Secondary polycythaemia
  - Nocturnal hypoxia (oxygen saturation less than 90% for more than 30% of the time)
  - Peripheral oedema
  - Pulmonary hypertension

- Current smoking is not an absolute contraindication to the use of LTOT. However smoking does create a significant fire and explosion hazard in the presence of oxygen

- Current smokers may also fail to gain much benefit in terms of life expectancy since their $FEV_1$ is continuing to decline at an accelerated rate

- COPD patients with chronic hypoxia may be dependent on a degree of hypoxia to drive their respiration (hypoxic respiratory drive). Too high a flow rate of oxygen will depress their respiratory drive, but too low a flow will fail to correct their hypoxia. The optimum flow rate of oxygen, therefore, needs to be determined by a specialist

- Patients and carers of patients on LTOT need clear advice on when to call a doctor in the event of worsening respiratory failure. They need to be able to recognise the symptoms – increasing drowsiness, mental confusion and headache – and need to understand the dangers of increasing the oxygen flow

- Once on LTOT, patients should have a specialist review at least annually to ensure that their oxygen needs are being met

## AMBULATORY OXYGEN THERAPY

- Ambulatory oxygen is delivered with portable oxygen systems, so it is suitable for patients on LTOT who regularly leave their homes and are well motivated

- Ambulatory oxygen is also used to improve exercise tolerance in those COPD patients who experience drops in oxygen saturation during exercise, but are not significantly hypoxic at rest

- Until the changes in oxygen prescribing due to come into force in late 2005, the use of ambulatory oxygen is severely limited by a lack of availability of suitable delivery systems on prescription

### Patient assessment

Under the new arrangements, assessment will be carried out by a specialist able to determine whether:

- There is a significant drop in oxygen saturation on exercise

- Ambulatory oxygen results in improved exercise tolerance or reduces breathlessness

- The flow rate of oxygen keeps the oxygen saturation above 90%

## Short-burst home oxygen therapy

- Short-burst oxygen is widely prescribed and is one of the most expensive therapies for COPD
- It is generally given to relieve distressing breathlessness and improve exercise capacity
- Despite its cost and widespread prescription, research to support the use of oxygen in this way is lacking
- NICE recommends that short-burst oxygen therapy should:
  - Only be considered for patients who experience distressing breathlessness not relieved by other therapies
  - Only be continued if there is a documented improvement in breathlessness with its use
  - Be provided from cylinders
- The new oxygen prescribing arrangements mean that this will be the only form of oxygen therapy GPs are able to prescribe

### VITAL POINT

*❋ Before short-burst oxygen is prescribed, it is worth considering whether the patient may fit the criteria for long-term oxygen therapy. Referral for specialist assessment may be appropriate*

## OXYGEN DELIVERY SYSTEMS

The systems for oxygen delivery available on prescription were limited to:

- Oxygen concentrators
- F-sized cylinders for domiciliary use
- PD, DD and CD cylinders for portable and short-term use
- Small portable cylinders, oxygen conserving devices and liquid oxygen were not available on prescription

The changes to oxygen prescribing due to come into force in late 2005 mean:

- GPs will be able to prescribe F-sized cylinders for short-burst oxygen therapy only

- All other systems – including liquid oxygen, portable oxygen and conserving devices – will be available through specialist oxygen services, funded via unified PCT budgets
- These services will be responsible for assessment of patients, the prescription of the most appropriate oxygen delivery system and the long-term supervision of patients

## Oxygen concentrators

- An oxygen concentrator is an electrically powered 'molecular sieve' that takes in room air, removes the nitrogen and carbon dioxide and delivers almost 100% oxygen to the patient
- Oxygen concentrators and all necessary disposables (nasal cannulae, tubing etc) are supplied, installed and serviced by the supply company whose services are contracted by the health authority
- Oxygen supply companies provide patients with 24 hour cover for concentrator breakdown and give valuable supervision, support and advice to patients and their carers. The cost of the electricity needed to run the concentrator is reimbursed directly to the patient
- The concentrator is placed in a suitable position in the patient's home (usually the hall) and oxygen is delivered through up to 50 metres of tubing. This allows the patient to mobilise throughout the home
- Concentrators are low-flow devices that don't contain a reservoir of oxygen. They represent a lower fire or explosion hazard than liquid oxygen or oxygen cylinders, but they should still be used with care

## VITAL POINTS

* *Oxygen concentrators are the most cost effective method of delivering LTOT*
* *The use of F-sized cylinders for LTOT delivery increases the cost tenfold*
* *If 2 or more oxygen cylinders are being prescribed per month the patient should be referred for assessment by a specialist*

## Oxygen cylinders (compressed gas)

- F-sized cylinders contain 1,360 litres of compressed oxygen, sufficient for 10–11 hours of oxygen at 2 l/minute
- PD cylinders are small enough to put into a car, but are generally too heavy for a patient with chronic lung disease to carry around
- DD and CD cylinders are the same size as the PD cylinder but, because of changes to the material and construction of the cylinder, contain more oxygen and are lighter
- Trolleys are available that enable patients to move around with a DD or CD cylinder
- Small, portable oxygen cylinders have a short 'life' unless they are used with an oxygen conserving device

## Liquid oxygen

- Liquid oxygen can be supplied in a large reservoir tank for use at home from which a portable tank lasting 8–9 hours can be filled

### VITAL POINT

*❋ All oxygen systems constitute a fire and explosion hazard. Patients must be explicitly warned about the hazards of smoking and using oxygen around naked flames*

## Masks and nasal cannulae

- Masks deliver either a fixed or variable percentage of oxygen
- Nasal cannulae are preferred for home use as they are less obtrusive and the patient is able to eat and drink while using them
- Drying of the nasal mucosa can be a problem and cannulae can cause pressure sores across the cheeks and behind the ears – particularly in thin patients
- The percentage of oxygen delivered via nasal cannulae is a product of the flow rate through the cannulae and the patient's breathing rate. Oxygen delivery is therefore variable. This is not generally problematic when the patient is stable, but may be important during exacerbations when the patient is in respiratory failure

## VITAL POINT

\* *The use of petroleum based creams or gels to prevent or relieve pressure sores and dryness caused by nasal cannulae constitutes an explosive hazard. Use water-based creams*

## REFERENCES

Medical Research Council (1981) Long-term domiciliary oxygen therapy in chronic hypoxic cor pulmonale complicating chronic bronchitis and emphysema. *Lancet*, 1: 681–686

National Collaborating Centre for Chronic Conditions (2004) Chronic obstructive pulmonary disease: National Clinical Guideline for management of chronic obstructive pulmonary disease in adults in primary and secondary care. *Thorax*, 59 (Suppl 1): 1–232. www.nice.org.uk/pdf/CG012_niceguideline.pdf

Nocturnal Oxygen Therapy Trial (NOTT) Group (1980) Continuous or nocturnal oxygen therapy in hypoxaemic chronic obstructive lung disease. A clinical trial. *Annals of Internal Medicine*, 93: 391–398

Royal College of Physicians (1999) *Domiciliary Oxygen Therapy Services: Clinical guidelines and advice for prescribers.* London: Royal College of Physicians

- Some people are better than others at maintaining their oxygen levels, despite severe COPD. Such individuals 'fight' hard to maintain oxygen levels by becoming very breathless. Suffering severe shortness of breath does not automatically mean that you need to be given oxygen and will benefit from it. You may in fact be maintaining your oxygen level by becoming breathless

- Why some people maintain oxygen levels and others don't is not understood

- As COPD progresses, it can cause you to have a chronically low level of oxygen in your blood. This puts a strain on your heart and will make you feel drowsy and unwell. Signs that this is happening include occasional swelling of your ankles, or a bluish tinge round your mouth or tongue

- Your doctor or nurse may measure your oxygen level during routine check-ups by clipping a machine called an oximeter to your finger. This is painless and takes a few seconds

- If your doctor thinks you would benefit from oxygen you will be sent to see a specialist. Assessment for oxygen will be done when you are well and will involve blood tests to check on the level of oxygen in your blood

- Oxygen is used in 2 ways. It is given to correct chronically low oxygen levels (long-term oxygen), or to relieve severe breathlessness and increase your ability to exercise (short burst oxygen)

- You should not use oxygen near naked flames. If you cook with gas it is not advisable to use your oxygen while you are cooking as there is a risk of fire or explosion

- If you are prescribed oxygen it is vital that you do not smoke while using it. Oxygen and cigarettes are an explosive combination. You risk severe burns or blowing yourself up if you do so

- When you are prescribed oxygen you should have regular check ups with a specialist, to check that your oxygen prescription is still meeting your needs

## LONG-TERM OXYGEN THERAPY (LTOT)

- LTOT aims to improve your quality of life and life expectancy. Being chronically short of oxygen can make you feel drowsy and unwell. LTOT can correct that and is also likely to reduce the number of times you need to be admitted to hospital

- LTOT must be used for at least 15 hours a day for you to gain any benefit. The more hours a day it is used the better. If you use it overnight, you can free up time during the day when you will not need to use it. This will allow you time to go out of the house without oxygen if you wish

- The flow rate of oxygen you should use will be prescribed. Usually this is between 2 and 4 litres per minute. It is very important NOT to turn up the flow rate without medical advice as this can make you worse

- The following are signs that you are either having too much or too little oxygen:
  - Severe headache
  - Mental confusion
  - Increasing drowsiness

- If you are experiencing any of these symptoms you should contact your doctor for advice. Do not be tempted to increase the flow rate of oxygen. More is not necessarily better

- LTOT is generally given with a machine called a concentrator. This runs on electricity and is about the size of a small fridge. It is plugged in at a convenient spot in your home, such as the hall. The engineer who fits the concentrator will advise you

- An oxygen concentrator can have up to 50 metres of tubing attached, so you can walk around your home while using it

- A specially qualified engineer will look after the concentrator for you and supply you with all the necessary equipment. The engineer will visit regularly to ensure that the concentrator is working properly and you are managing

- The engineer also checks the meter on the concentrator so you can be reimbursed for the electricity needed to run it. The running costs are sent to you directly, without delay

- You will also be given a telephone number that you can call night or day if the concentrator breaks down. An engineer will visit within 24 hours to deal with any problems

- You will not normally have to use an oxygen mask, unless you particularly want to

- Oxygen is given through nasal prongs. These are small tubes that sit just inside the nostrils and are attached to tubing that loops around the back of your ears and is fastened under your chin. These are quite discreet and you will be able to talk and eat normally while using them

- Nasal prongs can sometimes make your nose and throat dry. Make sure you drink plenty of fluids to overcome this problem

- Nasal prongs can make your nose sore. You will be advised on suitable creams to use. Do not use petroleum jelly or Vaseline

- Tubing across your cheeks and behind your ears can cause soreness. Special pieces of foam to fit around the tubing to relieve the pressure are available to reduce this problem

## PATIENT AND CARER INFORMATION
## SHORT-BURST OXYGEN THERAPY

- Oxygen from cylinders is sometimes prescribed to relieve breathlessness. This will generally be given to you by your GP in the form of oxygen cylinders

- Oxygen cylinders for short burst therapy will be too big to carry around and you will need to use it while sitting in a chair

- Ideally you should be assessed by a specialist before you are given oxygen for short burst use. You may actually need it for longer periods. A specialist assessment will ensure that you are being prescribed the most appropriate form of oxygen therapy

# 7 Living with COPD

COPD affects every area of a patient's life. Increasing breathlessness reduces the ability to perform every day activities and normal household tasks.

Relatives and carers are also affected by COPD. As the disease progresses they will often need to take on an increased domestic burden.

## BREATHLESSNESS ON EXERTION

- Patients with COPD often cope with breathlessness on exertion by avoiding activity. This leads to progressive loss of fitness and increasing breathlessness. Eventually they may be unable to get out of the house and will become socially isolated

- COPD patients and their relatives need to understand that breathlessness is not harmful and avoiding exercise makes things worse

- Simply telling a COPD patient that they are not doing any damage by getting breathless can be very reassuring

- All COPD patients should be encouraged to keep active and to take some form of exercise every day. Exercise that makes them moderately short of breath, but not incapacitated, is ideal

- Advice to take a regular walk at their own pace, or to climb stairs, fits in well with normal daily activity and is meaningful to patients

### VITAL POINT

*COPD patients who are becoming disabled by breathlessness should be referred for pulmonary rehabilitation, and every attempt made to motivate them to attend*

## Breathing control

- COPD patients who are becoming breathless tend to overuse the accessory muscles of respiration. These muscles are less efficient and tire more readily
- Teaching abdominal breathing, pursed-lip breathing and active cycle of breathing techniques can improve the efficiency of respiratory movements, reduce air trapping and assist expectoration
- If patients become breathless, they should be encouraged to adopt a position of relaxation, and practise abdominal or pursed-lip breathing until they recover

### VITAL POINT

❊ *Extreme breathlessness can provoke panic. Giving patients the tools to help them cope with breathlessness and avoid panic can be immensely beneficial*

## Energy conservation

- Most patients with COPD have to learn to pace themselves and avoid becoming overtired
- Activities that involve bending down and stretching up are usually most difficult
- Practical advice that makes everyday activities easier will be useful for most patients. Consider referring patients who have particular difficulty to an occupational therapist for assessment

### VITAL POINT

❊ *Enabling patients to continue with their normal activities helps them maintain independence and self esteem*

## Nutrition

- Weight loss is common in COPD and is associated with worsening prognosis

- Loss of lean muscle mass leads to worsening breathlessness on exertion; muscle fatigue often causes patients to stop activity before shortness of breath
- Breathlessness uses energy, so breathless patients have a high energy requirement
- Flattening of the diaphragms due to hyperinflation of the lungs, coupled with breathlessness can make eating a full meal difficult
- Breathlessness also makes shopping and cooking more difficult
- COPD does not only affect the lungs; it affects the whole body. Circulating inflammatory mediators and cytokines may also be responsible for weight loss in COPD
- Being overweight places additional strain on the cardiovascular and pulmonary systems. Such patients are likely to experience more breathlessness on exertion
- Measurement of Body Mass Index (BMI) should be a routine part of patient follow-up
- Patients with an abnormal BMI should be referred to a dietitian

## VITAL POINTS

*Dietary supplements can be helpful for underweight COPD patients, but they should not be prescribed without referral to a dietitian. Dietary supplements should not replace a normal diet*

*Patients who are receiving dietary supplements should also be advised to take exercise. This will help increase muscle mass and enable maximum benefit to be gained from dietary supplementation*

## PREVENTING EXACERBATIONS

### Vaccination

- Annual vaccination against influenza reduces mortality in COPD
- The vaccine is safe and effective
- Pneumococcal vaccination is also recommended for COPD patients, although evidence for its effectiveness in this patient group is lacking

## Avoiding exacerbations

- Advise patients to stay away from people (and babies) with colds, sore throats or sinus infections as much as possible
- Current smoking leads to more frequent exacerbations
- Staying away from smoky atmospheres and asking relatives and carers not to smoke is beneficial

- During episodes of poor air quality, COPD patients should be advised to stay indoors
- Avoiding places where there are a lot of exhaust fumes (eg underground carparks) may be helpful
- Air freshener sprays, scented candles, 'plug-in' air fresheners, strongly scented household cleaners, hairspray and perfume can irritate the airways of COPD patients and should be avoided
- Covering the mouth and nose with a scarf when the weather is cold and windy can be helpful

## Self-management plans

- Evidence for the benefit of giving COPD patients a self-management plan is contradictory at present. Further research is needed

- Until such time as research findings are available to give clear indication of what a COPD self-management plan should contain, the following recommendations from NICE provide a pragmatic approach:
  - Patients should be encouraged to take note of their usual symptoms when they are well, so that they perceive and can act on any changes
  - Symptoms that should prompt action include either an increase in sputum volume, or an increase in sputum purulence, or increasing breathlessness interfering with their ability to undertake their normal activities
- Should one or more of these symptoms occur, patients are advised to contact the doctor without delay
- Suitable patients may benefit from keeping a supply of antibiotics and oral corticosteroids at home so that they are able to initiate treatment promptly. They should be told to contact the doctor as soon as possible if they have initiated this therapy
- Self-management advice should be given verbally and written down for patients' reference

## TRAVEL

### Travel within the UK

- COPD patients should be encouraged to register with services that help them to remain mobile, socially interactive and 'normal'. Social isolation is a significant problem that should be overcome whenever possible
- Patients who are unable to walk more than 100 metres should be encouraged to apply for a 'blue (formally orange) badge' for their car. This will enable them to park close to their destination
- Registering as disabled with the local authority allows access to schemes such as 'Shopmobility' and 'Dial-a-ride'
- With forward planning, COPD patients planning travel overland within the UK are unlikely to experience significant problems
- Travel agents and local tourist information offices can provide information about accommodation with disabled access
- Patients who are oxygen-dependent can have oxygen supplied at their final destination, given sufficient notice. Or they can sometimes take oxygen concentrators with them to use when they arrive

## Travel abroad

- Travel by sea or overland should not pose a problem for COPD patients who are not oxygen dependent and who do not use nebulisers
- 'Blue badges' are valid for use across Europe
- Portable nebulisers, that run on car cigarette lighters or have integral rechargeable batteries are available
- Oxygen-dependent patients may be able to borrow portable oxygen or take their concentrator with them on holiday – provided they have permission
- Travel insurance can be problematic. Although reciprocal health care arrangements throughout the European Union covers health care, the cost of repatriation and additional expenses are not covered

## Air travel

- Assistance with transport around the airport is relatively easy to arrange. Wheelchairs and 'buggies' are available at all airports to help disabled passengers get to and from aircraft
- Pressurised aircraft cabins reduce the concentration of oxygen in the atmosphere from 21% to 15%
- COPD patients who are unable to compensate for this drop in oxygen concentration are likely to become significantly hypoxic during flight
- The BTS has produced guidelines for assessment of 'fitness to fly'. Patients with a resting oxygen saturation of 92–95% at sea level may not require oxygen, providing they have no additional risk factors (hypercapnia, $FEV_1$ <50% predicted, lung cancer, restrictive lung disease caused by pulmonary fibrosis, chest wall deformity or neuromuscular disease, dependency on ventilator support, cerebrovascular or cardiac disease, or within 6 weeks of an exacerbation)
- Patients with a resting oxygen saturation of 92–95% with additional risk factors and those with saturation below 92% should be referred for specialist assessment prior to flight
- 'In-flight' oxygen will be necessary for some patients. Not all airlines will supply oxygen and charges vary widely

## PSYCHOSOCIAL AND SEXUAL DIFFICULTIES

- Breathlessness and productive cough are embarrassing. A wish to avoid embarrassment can prevent a COPD patient from leaving their home and can lead to social isolation

- Inability to perform everyday tasks can result in loss of role within the family and lowered self-esteem

- Social isolation, guilt at having smoked and caused the problem, low self-esteem and loss of role can lead to depression and anxiety

- Patients with severe COPD are 2.5 times more likely to suffer from clinical depression than other members of the population

- Financial difficulties can occur if patients are unable to work and have had to retire early

## Significant others

- Relatives and carers carry an increased burden and suffer stress and anxiety as well. Spouses, who are likely to be middle aged or elderly and may have health problems of their own, can face particular difficulties
- Relationship difficulties are common amongst COPD patients and their families. Sexual difficulties can add to relationship problems, anxiety and depression. Referral to a specialist counsellor may be appropriate
- Breathlessness can make sexual and loving relationships difficult. COPD patients may find practical advice about suitable positions helpful

### VITAL POINTS

\* *Relatives and carers may be able to get support and help from carer's associations or by joining a self-help group such as Breathe Easy*

\* *Referral for specialist psychosexual or relationship counselling may be appropriate for some patients*

\* *COPD is a multi-component problem that requires a multidisciplinary approach*

## REFERENCES

British Thoracic Society (2002) Managing patients with respiratory disease planning air travel: British Thoracic Society recommendations. *Thorax*, 57: 289–304

Chief Medical Officer (2003) *Update on Immunisation Issues*. PL/CMO/2003/4

Monninkhof EM, van der Valk P, van der Palen J et al (2003) Self-management education for patients with chronic obstructive pulmonary disease: a systematic review. *Thorax*, 58: 394–8

National Collaborating Centre for Chronic Conditions (2004) Chronic obstructive pulmonary disease: National Clinical Guideline for management of chronic obstructive pulmonary disease in adults in primary and secondary care. *Thorax*, 59 (Suppl 1): 1–232. www.nice.org.uk/pdf/CG012_niceguideline.pdf

## BREATHLESSNESS WITH ACTIVITY

- Breathlessness with activity is a common symptom of COPD. Although it can be distressing it is not harming you. Indeed, getting moderately breathless on a regular basis is actually beneficial

- Regular exercise helps to keep your heart healthy and maintains the strength of your muscles. The more you keep doing, the more you are able to do, the longer you are able to keep active and the less breathless you will be

- You don't need to join a gym or use any special exercise equipment. Simple daily activity, such as taking a walk at your own steady pace or stair climbing, is helpful

- When you start to take exercise start slowly and build up the amount you do gradually. You should aim to eventually take 20–30 minutes exercise that makes you a little short of breath at least 4 times a week

- If you find your COPD is slowing you down and preventing you from normal activities, ask you doctor or nurse about pulmonary rehabilitation. This is a supervised exercise programme that would be helpful to you

## BREATHING EXERCISES

- If you become very breathless, try pursed-lip breathing to help you relax and regain control:
  - Relax your neck and shoulder muscles
  - Inhale slowly through your nose for a count of two
  - Purse your lips and breathe out gently through your lips to a count of four or more
  - Always breathe out for longer than you breathed in and always breathe out gently
- You may also find the following positions helpful for getting your breath back and relaxing:
  - Sit down, resting your forearms on your thighs. Keep your back straight and relax your neck and shoulder muscles

- Stand and lean backwards against a wall, relaxing your neck and shoulders
- Stand and lean your folded arms on a suitable height surface – such as a mantelpiece. Lean forward onto your arms and relax your neck and shoulders

- Abdominal breathing can help reduce breathlessness and improve the efficiency of your breathing. Practise this as follows, so that it becomes a habit:
  - Sit in a comfortable position and relax your neck and shoulder muscles
  - Place one hand on your chest and one on your tummy
  - Relax your tummy muscles and inhale slowly through your nose to the count of two. The hand on your chest should stay still and you should feel the hand on your tummy move outwards
  - Tighten your tummy muscles and exhale to the count of four. You should feel the hand on your tummy move inward while the hand on your chest stays still

- If you have difficulty clearing phlegm from your chest, the active cycle of breathing is an exercise you may find helpful:
  - Sit comfortably and take three to five slow deep breaths using pursed-lip and abdominal breathing
  - Take a normal breath in, then squeeze your chest and tummy muscles and force the breath out with your mouth open, making a 'huff' sound
  - Go back to pursed-lip and abdominal breathing
  - You may need to repeat this, with rests in between, up to 4 times

### *CONSERVING YOUR ENERGY*

- You will find that COPD prevents you doing all the things you used to do, or will slow you down. Pace yourself, so you can achieve all you want to do without getting overtired. Slow and steady will get you there in the end

- Make everyday life as easy for yourself as possible. Reaching up, bending down and carrying things are often difficult for people with COPD. Use a trolley with wheels to move things around, rather than carrying them

- Sit down as often as you can:
  - To prepare meals or wash up
  - To iron
  - To clean your teeth/shave, etc
- Place objects you use often at waist height, within easy reach. Try to avoid bending down. Use aids – eg a long handled gripper for reaching items on high shelves or picking things up off the floor
- If towelling yourself after a bath or shower is tiring, try wrapping yourself in a towelling robe instead
- If climbing in and out of a bath is difficult, consider showering

## HEALTHY EATING

- There is increasing evidence that eating a healthy diet with plenty of fresh fruit and vegetables is good for your lungs
- If you find eating a large meal leaves you feeling bloated and breathless, try eating smaller meals more often
- Eating healthy snacks between meals can help maintain your food intake if eating a full meal is difficult for you
- Quick, easy to prepare recipes make cooking for yourself easier
- Consider cooking more than you need when you are feeling well and freezing the surplus for days when you don't feel so good
- If you are overweight, try to reduce your weight. Carrying excess puts a strain on your heart and makes you more breathless
- If you are underweight, your doctor or nurse may suggest you see a dietitian or take some dietary supplements. These are intended to supplement a good diet, not replace it
- Sensible exercise will help you to get the most benefit from supplements, in terms of rebuilding lost muscle
- If you are using oxygen, use it while you are eating. This will reduce the amount of breathlessness you experience during meals.
- If eating makes you breathless, use your bronchodilator before meals. If you are very breathless, soft foods (eg mashed potato, fish, thick soup or purée) will be easier and less tiring to eat
- Bloating can be a problem and avoiding foods that produce excess gas, such as cabbage, or fizzy drinks can be helpful

- Make sure you drink enough. This will help to keep phlegm thin and easy to cough up, will help prevent constipation and keep your kidneys functioning well

## BAD ATTACKS AND CHEST INFECTIONS

- Flu can make you seriously ill if you have COPD. Vaccine is available every year at your doctor's surgery at the start of October. It is safe and effective – make sure you have your shot

- You should also be vaccinated against a type of pneumonia, caused by a germ called pneumococcus. This injection need only be given every 10 years. This is also safe and will not make you ill

- People with COPD are more prone to colds and viral infections. Try to avoid people of all ages who have colds, sore throats and sinus infections. Explain to friends and family that catching a cold could make you ill; ask them not to visit if they are unwell

- Smoking makes you prone to infection, as well as making your COPD worse. Your doctor or nurse will be happy to give you advice and support to help you stop. Ask your friends and family not to smoke around you

- Strong smells, such as household cleaners, scented candles and air-fresheners, or perfumes and air sprays can make you cough or feel breathless. They are best avoided

- Try to avoid areas where there are a lot of car exhaust fumes. Cold weather can also make you feel worse and staying indoors in the warm on very cold days, or wearing a scarf around your nose and mouth if you have to go out, may be helpful

- Be aware of how you feel normally. This will help you to recognise the early signs of an attack, so that you can take action to stop yourself from getting worse

- Early signs of an attack include:
  - More breathlessness than usual
  - More coughing
  - Producing more phlegm than usual or a change in the colour of your phlegm from grey/white to yellow or green
  - A sore throat
  - Feeling generally unwell

- If you notice any of these symptoms do not ignore them. Contact your doctor or nurse as prompt treatment may prevent a really serious attack
- If you are more breathless than usual, take your reliever inhaler more frequently. This is quite safe and will make you feel better
- If you have been given tablets to keep at home, make sure you have written instructions about when and how you should take them. If you need to start them let your doctor know as soon as possible

## *TRAVEL AND HOLIDAYS*

- If you are finding it difficult to get about, consider asking to be registered as disabled with your local authority. This will entitle you to a 'blue badge' parking sticker which can be used in your own car and by anybody else who drives you around
- Registering as disabled will also enable you to use any schemes such as 'Dial-a-ride' or 'Shopmobility' that are available in your area. These schemes are there to help you get out and about, which makes you less likely to become 'low' or depressed
- You can take holidays if you have COPD, but plan ahead:
  - If you use oxygen you will need to ask your doctor to arrange for an oxygen supply at your holiday destination
  - If you are planning air travel discuss this with your doctor before you book your holiday
- Some people with COPD need to use oxygen during a flight and your doctor may need to refer you to the hospital for assessment. If you use oxygen at home you will need to be assessed to determine how much oxygen you will need during the flight
- Travel insurance can be difficult. Remember that, although there are reciprocal health care arrangements throughout the EU, the cost of getting you back to the UK if you are ill, and additional expenses incurred because of illness are not covered
- The British Lung Foundation post helpful, up to date information about travel and holidays on their website (see page 109). They will be able to give you advice about how much airlines charge for oxygen during flight, which insurance companies will provide cover and which travel agents specialise in holidays for people with your particular health problems

## DEPRESSION AND ANXIETY

- It is not unusual for people living with COPD to get 'down' and depressed about their condition at times. Feeling angry and frustrated is natural and nothing to be ashamed about

- Discussing these feelings with your partner, family or carer can be helpful and will help them to understand how you are feeling

- If you are depressed or anxious you will be less able to cope with the daily difficulties of living with COPD. If your doctor suggests you might benefit from counselling or antidepressant medicines do listen. Accepting help can be a sign of strength

## LOVING RELATIONSHIPS

- Breathlessness can make sexual activity difficult, and this can impact on other aspects of your relationship too. If you are experiencing problems, you may find the following positions (also suitable for same sex couples) helpful:
  - Side by side, face to face
  - On the side with the man behind
  - Woman on top
  - Woman on the edge of the bed with the man kneeling on the floor in front

- Use your reliever inhaler before you start. You may also want to go and clear any phlegm first. Some people may prefer to avoid sex in the morning as this is when their cough is worse

- If you normally use oxygen, use it during lovemaking as it will help with breathlessness. Nasal cannulae should not get in the way

- None of the medicines used to treat your COPD affect your sex drive or your ability to have intercourse. However, it is normal for your sex drive to decline a little as you get older. It will take longer to achieve an erection and reaching orgasm will be slower

- If you are experiencing particular difficulties, do talk to your doctor. There are a number of things that can be done to help

- Bear in mind that sexual intercourse is not the only way of being intimate with your partner. Simple touching and closeness helps you both feel loved and special

# 8 Exacerbations

An exacerbation is:

*'A sustained worsening of the patient's symptoms from his or her usual stable state that is beyond normal day-to-day variations, and is acute in onset. Commonly reported symptoms are worsening breathlessness, cough, increased sputum production and change in sputum colour. The change in these symptoms often necessitates a change in medication.'* (NICE 2004)

Patients admitted to hospital with exacerbations of COPD account for 12.5% of all acute medical admissions. As the disease progresses they become more frequent, and are important for the following reasons:

- They are disabling and disruptive for patients and are often slow to resolve. Frequent exacerbations result in an accelerated decline in patients' health related quality of life
- Frequent exacerbations increase the rate of lung function decline and worsen prognosis
- They are expensive. Exacerbations account for a significant proportion of the total cost of caring for COPD
- Of the patients admitted to hospital with an exacerbation of COPD, 34% will be readmitted and 14% will have died within 3 months

## VITAL POINT

*\* Prevention and appropriate management of exacerbations of COPD is a key priority*

## CAUSES OF EXACERBATIONS OF COPD

In 30% of cases the cause of an exacerbation cannot be identified. Known causes include:

- Infections:
  - Viruses – rhinovirus (common cold), influenza, parainfluenza, coronavirus, adenovirus, respiratory syncitial virus (RSV)
  - Bacteria – *C. pneumoniae, H. influenzae, S. pneumoniae, M. catarrhalis, Staph. aureus* and *P. aeruginosa*
- Pollution:
  - Nitrogen dioxide
  - Particulates
  - Sulphur dioxide
  - Ozone

## SYMPTOMS OF EXACERBATIONS

The symptoms and severity of symptoms is extremely variable. There is no single defining symptom but the following are common:

- Increasing breathlessness
- Increasing cough and sputum production

Other presenting symptoms of COPD exacerbations include:

- Increased sputum purulence
- 'Colds' and/or sore throat
- Increased wheeze
- Reduced exercise tolerance
- Increased fatigue and general malaise
- Fluid retention and ankle oedema

Symptoms of a severe exacerbation include:

- Severe breathlessness
- Increased respiratory rate
- Pursed-lip breathing (unless this is habitual for this patient)
- Accessory muscle use at rest
- Acute mental confusion and/or drowsiness
- New onset of peripheral oedema or cyanosis
- Marked reduction in ability to carry out normal activities, or being confined to bed

## DIFFERENTIAL DIAGNOSIS

Many other conditions can present with similar symptoms to an exacerbation of COPD. These need to be considered and excluded:

- Pneumonia
- Pneumothorax
- Pulmonary embolism
- Pleural effusion
- Pulmonary oedema/left ventricular failure
- Lung cancer

## ASSESSING THE NEED FOR ADMISSION

The decision to admit a patient with an exacerbation of COPD is complex and involves consideration of a variety of social factors as well as the severity of the exacerbation.

| Indicators | Treat at home | Admit |
|---|---|---|
| Able to cope/support at home | Yes | No |
| Social circumstances | Good | Poor/lives alone/ not coping |
| General condition | Good | Poor |
| Significant co-morbidity (cardiac disease, diabetes) | No | Yes |
| Breathlessness | Mild | Severe |
| Level of activity | Normal | Reduced/ confined to bed |
| Acute confusion | No | Yes |
| Rapid onset of exacerbation | No | Yes |
| Cyanosed | No | Yes |
| Using LTOT | No | Yes |
| Worsening oedema | No | Yes |
| Abnormally drowsy | No | Yes |

The greater the number of indicators for hospital admission the more likely the need for management in hospital.

## DRUG THERAPY FOR EXACERBATIONS

### Bronchodilators

- Increased breathlessness is a key feature of an exacerbation. First line treatment is to increase the dose, or regularity of use, of short-acting bronchodilators
- Both normal hand-held inhalers and nebulisers are effective. There is no significant advantage of nebulisers over increased doses via hand-held inhaler
- When patients are very short of breath, large volume spacers may be helpful

- The choice of delivery system should depend on the dose of drug used, the ability of the patient to use the device and the available resources for supervision of drug administration
- Compressed air should be used to power nebulisers in a community setting. Most nebulisers require 6–8 l/min of flow to produce appropriate sized particles. A domiciliary oxygen cylinder can only produce 4 l/min; insufficient to power a nebuliser, unless fitted with a high flow regulator valve
- The respiration of a COPD patient dependent on a hypoxic respiratory drive (see page 107) may be suppressed by 6–8 litres of oxygen a minute

## Oral corticosteroids

- Short courses of oral corticosteroids have been found to be effective in:
  - Reducing the length of an exacerbation
  - Prolonging the time between exacerbations
  - Shortening the length of hospital stay in hospitalised patients
- They should be considered for:
  - All patients requiring hospital admission
  - Patients being managed at home where significant increases in the level of breathlessness interferes with daily activities
- Current recommendations from NICE are for oral prednisolone 30 mg daily, taken as a single morning dose for 7–14 days. Prolonged treatment over 2 weeks duration confers no significant benefit and increases the incidence of side effects
- A short course of oral corticosteroids of up to 2 weeks duration can be stopped abruptly. Tapering of the dose is not necessary unless the patient is on maintenance oral corticosteroids or has received frequent short courses. Guidance on this issue can be found in the *British National Formulary*
- Osteoporosis prophylaxis may be required for patients needing frequent short courses of oral corticosteroids

## Antibiotics

- Antibiotics should be used if the sputum becomes purulent
- It is not necessary to take sputum samples before initiating antibiotics
- The choice of antibiotic should depend on the guidance issued by the local microbiology service. First line antibiotics, such as amoxicillin, erythromycin and tetracycline, are usually effective

## OXYGEN THERAPY DURING EXACERBATIONS

- COPD patients with severe breathlessness during an exacerbation who need to be admitted to hospital are often given oxygen while waiting for an ambulance, during transport to the hospital and while being assessed in the hospital, with the aim of preventing life-threatening hypoxia

- Oxygen saturation should be measured and oxygen therapy commenced at 40%. The percentage of oxygen should be titrated upwards to keep saturation above 90%, and downwards if saturation rises above 93–94% or the patient becomes drowsy

## PREVENTING EXACERBATIONS

- All patients should be encouraged to have an annual influenza vaccination and should also be offered pneumococcal vaccination every 10 years

- Patients who experience 2 or more exacerbations a year should be given a long-acting bronchodilator (either beta2 agonist or anticholinergic), since their use is associated with a reduction in exacerbation rate
- COPD patients whose $FEV_1$ is less than 50% of predicted value who experience 2 or more exacerbations a year should be considered for long-term inhaled corticosteroids since they are associated with a reduced exacerbation rate
- Combination inhalers of long-acting beta2 agonist and inhaled corticosteroids may have a greater effect than either agent on its own. They are licensed for use in COPD
- Patients should be encouraged to be aware of their normal symptoms so that they can recognise the early warning signs of an exacerbation and report them to their doctor
- Self-management plans, written and verbal, with or without the provision of 'stand by' courses of antibiotics and oral corticosteroids, should be given to COPD patients who have regular exacerbations
- COPD patients should be encouraged to seek help early in the course of an exacerbation and not to wait until they are experiencing severe difficulty

## REFERENCES

Niewoehner DE, Erbland ML, Dupree RH et al (1999) Effect of systemic glucocorticoids on exacerbations of chronic obstructive pulmonary disease. *New England Journal of Medicine*, 340, 1941–1947

National Collaborating Centre for Chronic Conditions (2004) Chronic obstructive pulmonary disease: National Clinical Guideline for management of chronic obstructive pulmonary disease in adults in primary and secondary care. *Thorax*, 59 (Suppl 1): 1–232

Roberts CM, Lowe D, Bucknall CE et al (2002) Clinical audit indicators of outcome following admission to hospital with acute exacerbations of chronic obstructive pulmonary disease. *Thorax*, 57: 137–141

Turner MO, Patel A, Ginsburg S, Fitzgerald JM (1997) Bronchodilator delivery in acute airflow obstruction. A meta-analysis. *Archives of Internal Medicine*, 157: 1736–1744

- All too often, crisis intervention and hospital admission are what patients with end-stage COPD can expect
- As a method of delivering high quality care, this approach is both expensive and ineffective
- Recurrent themes to emerge from qualitative studies of dying with COPD include:
  - ◆ Very poor quality of life for patients and carers
  - ◆ Little contact with community services such as district nursing, social work or day care
  - ◆ Poor, or delayed provision of home adaptations (eg showers, stair lifts, grab rails) that would improve patients' independence and lessen the burden on carers
  - ◆ Poor provision of information. Few bereaved relatives realised that COPD might be terminal
- The natural history of COPD can extend over many years and determining when an individual has reached 'end-stage' is extremely difficult. Many patients struggle on with appalling lung function and symptoms, but a stable clinical state
- Choosing the right moment to discuss issues of prognosis, ventilation and advanced directives is not easy
- GPs and practice nurses often have the advantage of knowing the patient and their family over many years and may be in a better position than secondary care staff to raise these difficult issues. However, although 82% of patients wanted their GP to discuss their prognosis, 37% of GPs admitted that they found it difficult to raise the issue and 30% left it to patients or their relatives to raise the subject

## WHAT PATIENTS WANT

- Research in palliative care and end-of-life is difficult and encroaches on sensitive areas. Most of what little research there is comes from the USA

- When extrapolating the results of this to a UK population, cultural differences need to be considered:
  - 89% of patients want to learn more about advanced directives
  - 69% want explicit information about intubation and mechanical ventilation
  - Although 99% of patients said that they would find such discussions acceptable only 19% had already discussed advanced directives and only 15% had discussed ventilation
  - 98% of the small number of patients who had discussed end of life issues had raised the subject themselves

## Features of end-stage COPD

- Severe symptoms include:
  - Unremitting breathlessness – even at rest. Such patients are often dependent on oxygen and have difficulty talking and eating
  - An inability to perform everyday tasks (eg washing, shaving) without help. Many patients are effectively chair or bed bound and heavily dependent
  - Overwhelming fatigue
- Before determining that a patient has reached the terminal phase of their disease it is important that:
  - Bronchodilator therapy has been optimised
  - Corticosteroid therapy has been tried
  - Appropriate oxygen has been prescribed
- Frequent hospital admissions mean that:
  - The 'revolving door' patient, with increasingly frequent and prolonged admissions, is common
  - Patients fail to derive benefit from hospital admission
  - Many patients will have been ventilated during a previous admission

## Symptom relief in the end stages of COPD

- Breathlessness can be particularly distressing for patients and their families
- If optimal bronchodilator therapy fails to relieve the symptoms, opioids can be considered. Although these will result in some degree of respiratory suppression, the benefit of relieving distressing symptoms may outweigh the risks at this stage of the disease

- Benzodiazepines, tricyclic antidepressants, major tranquillisers and oxygen may also be helpful

## Palliative care

- Palliative care is 'the active, total care of patients and their families by a multi-professional team when the patient's disease is no longer responsive to curative treatments'
- It is similar to, but distinct from 'terminal care'
- The role of the palliative care team in cancer care is well established, and there is now increasing recognition of the need to extend team roles to encompass non-malignant disease as well

### VITAL POINTS

❋ *Ensure that all standard forms of management have been tried before end-stage COPD is diagnosed*

❋ *Patients with end-stage COPD, and their families and carers should have access to palliative care services, including hospice care*

## Advanced directives ('Living Wills')

- Advanced directives are not supported by legislation, but they are recognised in case law and doctors are expected to comply with them
- They are a statement of a patient's wishes regarding which medical interventions they do not wish to receive
- The wording of an advanced directive is best kept as simple as possible. It cannot cover every situation that may arise, but should convey the spirit of the patient's wishes
- In order for an advanced directive to be valid it must have been discussed with a doctor and include:
  - The patient's name and address
  - A clear statement of their wishes – general or specific
  - The name and address of the GP
  - The patient's signature and the signature of a witness
  - The date

- ◆ The name and address of the patient's health care proxy (if appropriate)
- ▪ The doctor should mark the notes and ask the patient to sign them
- ▪ A copy of the directive should be filed in the notes and reviewed annually

## VITAL POINT

✳ *Relatives and carers must be actively involved in discussion of advanced directives if patients' wishes for their end-of-life care are to be fulfilled*

### Artificial ventilation

- ▪ Non-invasive ventilation (NIV) is effective and the treatment of choice for COPD patients with hypercapnic respiratory failure that is not responding to other treatment during an exacerbation
- ▪ NIV is delivered via a tightly fitting nasal or facial mask, enabling patients to receive ventilation without sedation and intubation
- ▪ NIV is usually available on the wards or in a high dependency unit and patients may not need to be admitted to ITU
- ▪ Invasive ventilation via an endotracheal tube will necessitate sedation and admission to ITU. Weaning from ventilation can be difficult and the patient is at risk of the complications of long-term sedation and intubation
- ▪ NIV has served to make 'end-stage' COPD more difficult to determine. It has enabled patients with very severe COPD who are unsuitable for invasive ventilation and ITU care to be effectively treated for acute respiratory failure
- ▪ Before NIV is commenced, decisions must be made about what to do in the event of failure. For some patients NIV will be the 'ceiling' of treatment; for others transfer to ITU and invasive ventilation may be an option. Involvement of relatives and carers is vital. An advanced directive can simplify this difficult decision
- ▪ Ventilation and life support should be discussed when the patient is in a stable condition

## PRACTICAL SUPPORT

- Caring for a terminally ill relative is exhausting and distressing. Many carers are elderly, and may have health problems of their own
- Encourage patients and carers to apply for all the benefits they are entitled to. They may require help in completing complex claim forms
- Registering as disabled enables access to schemes that can make the carer's life easier, as well as helping the patient to get out of the house
- Social services can arrange an occupational therapy assessment. The provision of aids that lighten the burden of care and enable the patient to maintain some degree of independence can be very beneficial. The provision of a wheelchair, while not appropriate at an earlier stage, may enable some degree of mobility and social interaction
- Respite care may become necessary

### VITAL POINT

> \* *Family support is the greatest asset a patient can have. Every effort should be made to involve family members, and ensure that they get as much help and support as possible*

### REFERENCES

British Thoracic Society (2002) Guidelines on non-invasive ventilation for acute respiratory failure. *Thorax*, 57: 192–211. www.brit-thoracic.org.uk/docs/NIV.pdf

Elkington H, White P, Higgs R, Pettinari CJ (2001) GPs' views of discussions of prognosis in severe COPD. *Family Practice*, 18: 440–444

Heffner JE, Fahy B, Hilling L, Barbieri C (1996) Attitudes regarding advance directives among patients in pulmonary rehabilitation. *American Journal of Respiratory and Critical Care Medicine*, 154: 1735–1740

National Collaborating Centre for Chronic Conditions (2004) Chronic obstructive pulmonary disease: National Clinical Guideline for management of chronic obstructive pulmonary disease in adults in primary and secondary care. *Thorax*, 59 (Suppl 1): 1–232

Rhodes P (1999) Focus on palliative care. Palliative care: the situation of people with chronic obstructive pulmonary disease. *British Journal of Community Nursing*, 4: 131–136

# PATIENT AND CARER INFORMATION

- Unfortunately there is no cure for COPD. Modern treatments can help you to stay as well as possible for as long as possible, but eventually you may come to a stage when you become terminally ill as a result of your COPD

- Although your symptoms will become worse (and in the severe and terminal phases can be very distressing for you and your family) it is important to remember that there are things that can be done to help

- Be sure to discuss any concerns or fears you have about the future with your doctor or nurse. They may not be able to be precise about what exactly will happen or when, but it will be helpful to you and those who look after you to discuss this together. This will help ensure that you are looked after in the way that you and your family wish

- Living with severe COPD can be difficult. You and your family need to apply for all the support you are entitled to. You will have earned it and should not feel embarrassed about asking for it. Information is available from Citizens Advice and the Benefits Agency

- Your doctor may suggest that an occupational therapist visit you to see if there are any aids that will make your daily life easier

- If your COPD is severe, there may be times when you need to be admitted to hospital. If your breathing is so bad that you cannot get enough oxygen into your body, you may need to go onto a life support machine (a ventilator). This will support your breathing while you recover from the attack

- There are two main ways of using a ventilator:
  - You may need to be sedated and given paralysing drugs so that a tube can be passed through your mouth and down into your windpipe. If this method is used you will need to go into an intensive care unit and will not be fully aware of what is going on around you
  - The method used most often for people with COPD is called non-invasive, or nasal ventilation. You will be fitted with a tightly fitting mask that will fit over your nose, or over your nose and mouth. The ventilator will then be used to 'boost' your own

breathing. You will be conscious and you will be able to remove the mask if you need to cough, talk, eat or drink. You will not necessarily need to go to intensive care

- If your breathlessness becomes very distressing, there are treatments that can help. Your doctor may refer you to a team of professionals who specialise in caring for people coming to the end of their lives. They will know how best to relieve your breathlessness, and will make you as comfortable as possible

# 10 Structuring care in general practice

- The majority of patients with mild and moderate COPD can be cared for in a primary care setting. As the disease progresses the need for secondary care services is likely to increase
- Good communication between primary and secondary care is essential if the patient is to experience 'seamless' care

## GENERAL MEDICAL SERVICES CONTRACT (nGMS)

- nGMS has raised the profile of COPD in primary care
- There are currently some areas of conflict between the requirements of nGMS and the evidence based NICE guideline for COPD
- The Quality and Outcome Framework for chronic disease management in nGMS offers a sliding scale of payment to practices according to their performance:
  - ◆ The practice can produce a register of patients with COPD
  - ◆ 25–90% of newly diagnosed patients (since April 2003) have had their diagnosis confirmed with spirometry AND reversibility testing
  - ◆ 25–90% of all the patients on the COPD register in whom the diagnosis has been confirmed by spirometry AND reversibility testing
  - ◆ 25–90% of COPD patients have had their smoking status recorded in the previous 15 months
  - ◆ 25–90% of those patients who continue to smoke whose notes contain a record that smoking cessation advice, or referral to a specialist smoking cessation service has been offered in the previous 15 months
  - ◆ 25–70% of patients have had their $FEV_1$ recorded in the previous 27 months

- 25–90% of patients using inhalers have had their technique checked in the previous 15 months
- 25–85% of patients have had influenza vaccine in the previous 15 months

## KEEPING A REGISTER: FINDING PATIENTS

- COPD is known to be under diagnosed. Many patients with mild or moderate COPD will either be unknown to their doctor or treated for recurrent chest infections or asthma
- One study suggests that the true prevalence of COPD may be as high as 11% of over 45-year-olds
- Follow up those current and ex-smokers who attend every winter with a chest infection, and offer spirometry
- Review the asthma register and perform spirometry on those patients who:
  - Are current or ex-smokers
  - Developed 'asthma' in middle age
  - Do not have a record of an objective diagnosis of asthma
  - Have a history which is more compatible with COPD than asthma (see page 25)
- Encourage smokers with a smoker's cough to attend for spirometry by putting a poster in the waiting room. The COPD consortium of The British Thoracic Society (see page 109) can provide these free of charge
- Routine screening of smokers with a spirometer is time-consuming but has a detection rate of 18%
- Smokers over the age of 35 years with chronic cough are a worthwhile group to target for spirometry (see page 21)

### VITAL POINT

*✳ The first step to improving the diagnosis rate of COPD is to think of it as a possibility in any current or ex-smoker, aged over 35, presenting with respiratory symptoms*

## Spirometry and reversibility testing

- Spirometry is essential for the accurate diagnosis of COPD
- Routine reversibility testing is not recommended in the NICE guideline, yet is included in nGMS
- Until the nGMS contract is reviewed in 2006, the following approach fulfils the requirements of nGMS and is in line with the evidence-based NICE guideline. When the history suggests COPD, the spirometry is obstructed and there are no features of asthma:
  - Treat the patient for COPD by putting them on a therapeutic trial of bronchodilators
  - Review after 4–6 weeks of treatment and tell the patient to take their bronchodilator before coming in to see you
  - Repeat the spirometry and compare it with the initial spirometry
  - Assess the patient's symptomatic response over the therapeutic trial
  - Reconsider the diagnosis of COPD if there is a 400 ml or more improvement in the $FEV_1$ or the patient reports an unexpectedly good response to therapy
- The $FEV_1$ at the end of the trial can be recorded as a reversibility test for nGMS since it is a post bronchodilator recording
- A review of the spirometry and symptomatic response following initial diagnosis will ensure that asthma is not missed

## Smoking status and support to stop

- Smoking is the most important cause of COPD and quitting the only intervention that slows the progression of the disease
- See pages 30–39 for detailed advice about encouraging patients to stop smoking

## Monitoring lung function

- nGMS requires a record of $FEV_1$ only every 2 years. More frequent monitoring is recommended in the NICE guideline, so that patients losing lung function rapidly can be detected and referred for specialist assessment
- Patients with mild and moderate COPD should have their $FEV_1$ measured at least annually and those with severe COPD at least twice a year
- Patients who have lost >500 ml of $FEV_1$ over 5 years require specialist assessment

## Inhaler technique and vaccination

- Inhaler technique should be checked regularly
- Influenza vaccine is of proven benefit to COPD patients in reducing hospital admissions and mortality
- The vaccine is safe and well tolerated. The only contraindication is an allergy to egg
- COPD patients should be encouraged to have annual influenza vaccination and pneumococcal vaccination every 10 years (see page 71)

---

### VITAL POINTS

*\* nGMS provides an incentive to call and recall COPD patients in order to fulfil the requirements of the quality outcome framework*

*\* This consultation is an ideal opportunity to review areas not covered in nGMS, but recommended in the NICE guideline*

---

## ROUTINE REVIEW OF PATIENTS:
## NICE RECOMMENDATIONS

- Patients with mild and moderate COPD should be reviewed at least annually and those with severe disease at least twice a year

### Mild and moderate COPD

- Enquire how adequately therapy is controlling the patient's symptoms and assess the effects of each therapy. Consider intensifying therapy if this is inadequate
- Ask about exercise tolerance – is this worsening?
- Assess whether the patient feels functionally disabled. Consider referral for pulmonary rehabilitation
- Ask about the frequency of exacerbations. Consider intensifying therapy if there have been more than 2 exacerbations in the previous 12 months

- Consider whether the patient needs referral for a specialist opinion or specialist therapy services
- Assess smoking status and desire to quit
- Measure the $FEV_1$ and FVC, calculate the BMI and record the MRC Dyspnoea Score

### Severe COPD

In addition to the above:

- Look for signs of cor pulmonale
- Assess the patient's nutritional state
- Assess the psychological state. Are they anxious or depressed?
- Consider whether the patient needs Social Service or Occupational Therapy Services
- Measure the $FEV_1$ and FVC, the BMI and oxygen saturation and record the MRC Dyspnoea Score

## VITAL POINTS

* Call and recall of patients on the COPD register requires organisation. Systems are necessary to follow up non attenders

* Housebound patients with severe COPD may need home visits for routine review

### Organisational issues

- Consideration needs to be given to allocating sufficient time to review patients:
  - Dedicated clinics may ensure patients see an appropriate health professional equipped and trained to deliver quality care
  - Review during normal surgery hours may be more flexible for patients, but result in insufficient allocation of time
- A nurse-led service requires nurses to be appropriately trained and sufficiently supported by other members of the primary care team
- Patient group directions will be required for a nurse-led service to allow administration of bronchodilators, vaccinations etc

- A protocol for patient management is essential – agreed upon and followed by all members of the primary care team
- Clerical support will be needed for call and recall of patients
- Management templates/Read codes need to be agreed and standardised throughout the practice to enable accurate audit and collection of data for nGMS payment
- Clerical support for collection of audit and nGMS data may also be required
- Funds need to be allocated to the provision and maintenance of equipment (eg a spirometer, one-way or filter mouthpieces, a pulse oximeter)
- Mechanisms for easy referral of patients to other services (eg dietetics, physiotherapy, occupational therapy, social services) need to be considered

## VITAL POINT

*❊ COPD is a multi-component disease that requires the organisation of a seamless and efficient, multidisciplinary team approach*

## TRAINING ISSUES

- Health professionals responsible for managing the routine care of COPD patients need to be appropriately trained for this role
- Many primary care based nurses are taking on the long-term care of COPD patients. The more their involvement in COPD care and the higher their level of autonomy, the greater the level of training that is required

## AUDIT

Audit is necessary in order to claim nGMS payment but is also essential for highlighting problem areas early and ensuring that services continue to improve.

### Audit of process

The following are required for nGMS payment:

- Number of patients on the COPD register
- Percentage of newly diagnosed patients who have had the diagnosis confirmed by spirometry and reversibility
- Percentage of COPD patients who:
  - Have ever had spirometry and reversibility performed
  - Have had smoking status recorded
  - Continue to smoke, despite having been given advice to stop
  - Have had $FEV_1$ recorded in the previous 27 months
  - Have had their inhaler technique checked
  - Have had an influenza vaccination in the previous season

Other areas that may be helpful to look at include:

- Percentage of smokers and ex-smokers who have had spirometry measurements taken
- Percentage of COPD patients who have received pneumococcal vaccination

## Audit of outcome

Although a useful starting point, process audit does not provide information about the quality of care and whether care is having a beneficial impact on patients. It may be helpful to audit the following outcomes:

- Percentage of the practice population with a diagnosis of COPD (is this in line with the expected prevalence rate?)
- Percentage of COPD patients who continue to smoke (is this falling?)
- Percentage of patients who have a good inhaler technique (is this rising?)
- The number of emergency admissions for COPD
- The number of emergency GP consultations
- Percentage of COPD patients who have been offered or have undertaken a pulmonary rehabilitation programme

## REFERENCES

Letter from the Chief Medical Officer, the Chief Nursing Officer and the Chief Pharmaceutical Officer (2003) Update on Immunisation Issues. PL/CMO/2003/4

National Collaborating Centre for Chronic Conditions (2004) Chronic obstructive pulmonary disease: National Clinical Guideline for management of chronic obstructive pulmonary disease in adults in primary and secondary care. *Thorax*, 59 (Suppl 1), 1–232. www.nice.org.uk/pdf/CG012_niceguideline.pdf

National Health Service Confederation, British Medical Association (2003) *Investing in General Practice: The New GMS Contract*. www.bma.org.uk/ap.nsf/Content/NewGMScontract/$file/gpcont.pdf

Renwick DS, Connolly MJ (1996) Prevalence and treatment of chronic airways obstruction in adults over the age of 45. *Thorax*, 51(2): 164–168

van Schayck CP, Loozen JMC, Wagena E, Akkermans RP, Wesseling GJ (2002) Detecting patients at high risk of developing chronic obstructive pulmonary disease in general practice: a cross sectional case finding study. *British Medical Journal*, 324: 1370–1374

# Glossary

**Accessory muscles** Muscle groups (eg sternomastoids, abdominal muscles) that can be used to assist respiration when the main muscles of respiration, the diaphragms, are inadequate. Accessory muscle use at rest or on minimal exertion is a prominent feature of COPD

**Advanced directive** A formal statement of an individual's wishes about which medical interventions they do not want. They are not supported by legislation, but are recognised in case law and doctors are expected to follow them. To be valid they must be discussed with a doctor and must be signed and witnessed

**Aerobic exercise** Exercise to increase the efficiency of the heart and lungs in delivering oxygen to the tissues

**Allergens** Substances that produce an allergic reaction

**Alpha 1 antitrypsin** An enzyme in the blood that provides the lungs with some protection against the harmful effects of cigarette smoking. Congenital deficiency of this enzyme is associated with the development of severe emphysema at a young age

**Alveolar ducts** The air passages that lead directly into the alveoli

**Alveoli** Microscopic air sacs in the lungs, in which the exchange of oxygen and carbon dioxide between the atmosphere and the circulation takes place

**Ambulatory oxygen** Oxygen that can be used while the patient is walking about, including outside the home. It is delivered with portable oxygen systems

**Anticholinergic bronchodilator** A drug which dilates the airways by blocking the action of acetylcholine on the parasympathetic nerve endings in the lungs

**Anxiolytics** Drugs used to treat anxiety states

**Arterial blood gases** Measurement of the amount of oxygen and carbon dioxide dissolved in the plasma of an arterial blood sample, measured in kilopascals (kPa). Also allows assessment of the acidity or alkalinity of the blood (pH)

**Asthma** Chronic inflammatory condition of the airways, leading to widespread, variable airway obstruction that is reversible spontaneously or with treatment. Long-standing asthma can produce irreversible airway obstruction

**Atopy** Hereditary disposition to develop allergic (atopic) diseases including asthma, eczema, hay fever and chronic rhinitis. Associated with high levels of the antibody IgE

**Auscultation** Listening to the chest with a stethoscope

**Beta2 agonist bronchodilator** A drug which stimulates beta2 receptors of the sympathetic nervous system in the lungs, resulting in bronchodilation

**Beta-blocking medication** Drugs which block the beta receptors of the sympathetic nervous system. Used to treat high blood pressure and heart failure. Use with caution in patients with airflow obstruction

**Body Mass Index (BMI)** Relationship of body weight to height used to assess nutritional status. BMI = weight (in kg) divided by height (in metres) squared. Normal range is 20–25

**Bronchiectasis** Irreversible dilation of the bronchi as a result of bronchial wall damage, causing chronic cough and the production of mucopurulent sputum

**Bronchioles** Smaller branching airways, usually 2 mm or less in diameter; subdivisions of the bronchi

**Bronchomotor tone** The normal resting muscle tone of the airways

**Cachexia** Morbid weight loss, or extreme emaciation

**Cardiac arrhythmia** An abnormality in the regularity of the heartbeat, caused by a defect in the generation or conduction of electrical impulses in the heart

**Chronic bronchiolitis** *See* small airway disease

**Chronic bronchitis** The production of sputum on most days for at least 3 months, in at least 2 consecutive years

**Collagen** A connective tissue; deposition of collagen in the airway of a patient with asthma contributes to irreversible airway obstruction

**Co-morbidity** A state of suffering from two or more pathological conditions at the same time

**Cor pulmonale** Pulmonary hypertension and right ventricular hypertrophy occurring as a result of chronic lung disease. The main clinical signs are cyanosis, peripheral oedema, raised jugular venous pressure and liver enlargement

**Corticosteroids** Hormones produced by the adrenal glands. Synthetic forms are used to treat a wide variety of inflammatory conditions. They are taken orally in short courses to treat severe exacerbations of COPD. Inhaled corticosteroids are used long-term to prevent exacerbations in patients with moderate and severe COPD

**Cyanosis** Blueness of the skin due to hypoxia. This is a subjective clinical finding, but is generally apparent when the oxygen saturation falls below 85–90%

**Disability** The extent to which a patient's ability to function is affected by ill health

**Dyspnoea** Awareness of increased respiratory effort that is perceived as unpleasant or inappropriate

**Emphysema** A destructive process involving the alveoli and, in its severe form, the terminal bronchioles and alveolar ducts as well. Destruction of the alveolar wall results in disrupted gas exchange and loss of the natural elasticity of the lungs

**Emphysematous bullae** Large, cyst-like spaces in the lung that compress normal tissue

**Exacerbation** A sustained worsening of symptoms from the usual stable state that is acute in onset. Commonly reported symptoms include worsening breathlessness, cough, increased sputum production and change in sputum colour

**Fibrosis** Scarring or thickening of an organ or tissue by replacement of the original tissue with collagenous fibrous tissue

**Fixed airflow obstruction** Airflow obstruction that does not fully reverse even with intensive therapy

**Flow/volume trace** A graph produced by a spirometer in which flow rate (in litres/second) is plotted on the vertical axis and volume (in litres) is plotted on the horizontal axis

**Forced expiratory volume in one second (FEV$_1$)** The amount of air that can be exhaled in the first second of a forced blow from maximum inhalation

**Forced vital capacity (FVC)** The amount of air that can be exhaled from maximum inhalation to maximum exhalation using maximum effort

**Gas transfer (TLCO)** A test performed in a lung function laboratory, demonstrating the ability of the lungs to take up a small amount of carbon monoxide. It is a measure of how efficient the alveoli are at gas exchange

**Health status** A measure of the impact of disease on a patient's daily life and social and emotional well-being

**Hypertrophy** An abnormal increase in the size of an organ or tissue

**Hyperinflation** Enlargement of the lungs due to increased volumes of trapped air. This leads to flattening of the diaphragms and inefficient respiratory movements

**Hypoxia** Low levels of oxygen in the blood (ie below 10 kPa)

**Hypoxic respiratory drive** A stimulus to breath that is driven by low levels of oxygen. When patients with this abnormal drive are given high levels of oxygen the stimulus to breathe will be suppressed, resulting in worsening respiratory failure or respiratory arrest

**Jugular venous pressure (JVP)** An indirect (and not 100% reliable) method of assessing pressure in the right atrium. With the patient lying at a 45$^{o}$ angle observe the highest point of pulsation of the internal jugular vein. Take a horizontal line from this point and measure the distance from this line to the sternal angle. A normal jugular venous pressure is about 4 cm

**Lobectomy** Surgical excision of one or more lobes of the lung

**Long-term oxygen therapy (LTOT)** Oxygen used for 15 hours a day or more. It improves life expectancy in COPD patients with chronic hypoxia

**Metastases** Secondary, malignant tumours that have spread from the site of the original tumour to another organ

**Mucolytics** Drugs which reduce the viscosity (stickiness) of mucus

**Nebuliser** A device which atomises a drug solution into particles small enough to be inhaled and deposited in the peripheral airways of the lungs

**Neurotransmitter** A chemical released by a neuron that, by binding to neuron receptors, stimulates or inhibits them

**Nicotine replacement therapy (NRT)** A method of reducing nicotine withdrawal symptoms in smokers attempting to stop

**Osteoporosis** Demineralisation and atrophy of bone, associated with increased risk of fracture. It is most commonly seen in post menopausal women but is also associated with long-term, or frequent short courses of oral corticosteroid

**Oxygen concentrator** An electrically powered molecular 'sieve' that removes nitrogen and carbon dioxide from room air and delivers almost pure oxygen to the patient

**Oxygen conserving device** A device which delivers oxygen only when the patient inhales, thus reducing wastage of oxygen during exhalation and extending the use of portable oxygen systems

**Oxygen saturation** The percentage of haemoglobin saturated with oxygen, measured with a pulse oximeter. Normal oxygen saturation is over 95

**Peak expiratory flow (PEF)** The maximum flow rate that can be maintained over the first 10 milliseconds of a forced exhalation from a position of maximum inhalation using maximum effort

**Pneumonectomy** Surgical excision of a lung

**Polycythaemia** An abnormal increase in the number of red blood cells; can arise as a result of chronic hypoxia

**Pulmonary oedema** Extravasated fluid in the lungs; commonly a result of left ventricular failure

**Pulmonary hypertension** Abnormally high pressure within the blood vessels of the lungs

**Pulmonary rehabilitation** A programme of exercise and education aimed at reducing disability and improving health status in chronic respiratory disease

**Pulse oximetry** A simple, non-invasive method of measuring oxygen saturation

**Respiratory failure** Failure to maintain oxygenation, usually taken to mean failure to maintain oxygen levels at above 8 kPa

**Short-burst oxygen** Oxygen therapy prescribed on an 'as needed' basis for the relief of distressing breathlessness

**Shuttle walk test** A method of assessing exercise endurance. The patient walks between two cones 10m apart at a speed dictated by tape recorded 'bleeps'. The speed is incrementally increased until the patient can no longer keep up or is forced to stop because of breathlessness

**Small airway disease** Pathological changes to airways 2–5mm in diameter. These include occlusion of the airway with mucus, thickening of the muscle around the airway, oedema of the airway wall and fibrosis around the airway

**Smoking 'pack years'** Calculation of an individual's total cigarette exposure by multiplying the number smoked per day by number of years as a smoker, divided by 20

**Spirometry** Measurement of lung volumes and air flow rates with an instrument called a spirometer. It is essential in diagnosing COPD

**Terminal bronchiole** The smallest generation of airway, leading into the alveolar ducts

**Theophyllines** Methylxanthine bronchodilator drugs, now rarely used

**Therapeutic trial** A means of assessing response to drug treatment. This is the preferred method of determining which bronchodilators are most effective for an individual COPD patient

**Volume time trace** A graph produced by a spirometer in which volume (in litres) is plotted on the vertical axis and time (in seconds) is plotted on the horizontal axis

**Wheeze** A 'whistling' breath sound. COPD patients may notice it, or it can be heard with a stethoscope

# Useful addresses and contacts

## Training organisations

### Eduction for Health
The Athenaeum
10 Church Street
Warwick
CV34 4AB
Tel: 01926 493313
Fax: 01926 493224
Website: www.nrtc.org.uk
*Education for Health (incorporating the National Respiratory Training Centre and Heartsave) is an accredited institute of the Open University. It offers one day short courses, diploma level and degree level modular courses in a wide range of respiratory disorders and an MSc in respiratory care*

### Respiratory Education and Training Centres
Website: www.respiratoryetc.com
*Offers a range of one day training and diploma and degree level modules in respiratory disease*

### The British Thoracic Society
17 Doughty Street
London
WC1N 2PL
Tel: 020 7831 8778
Website: www.brit-thoracic.org.uk
*Seeks to preserve and protect public health by the provision of information in matters concerning respiratory and associated disorders and how they might be prevented*

## Patient information and support organisations

### British Lung Foundation
73–75 Goswell Road
London
EC1V 7ER
Tel: 020 7688 5555
Fax: 020 7831 5556
Website: www.britishlungfoundation.com
Helpline: 0845 8505020
open Mon–Fri 10 a.m.–6 p.m.
*A charity working to support people with respiratory disease by raising money for research, campaigning for better health service provision for respiratory disease, providing useful information for patients on a range of topics and facilitating and supporting the development of Breathe-Easy patient self-help groups. A telephone helpline for patients is also available*

### Quit: (Smoking Quitlines)
England: 0800 00 22 00
Northern Ireland: 028 90 663 281
Scotland: 0800 84 84 84
Wales: 0800 169 0 169
*For help with trying to stop smoking*

*Have you found **Vital COPD** useful and practical? If so, you may be interested in other books from Class Publishing.*

### Chronic Obstructive Pulmonary Disease in Primary Care
THIRD EDITION            £29.99
*Dr David Bellamy and Rachel Booker*

This clear and helpful resource manual addresses the management requirements of GPs and practice nurses. In this book, you will find guidance, protocols, plans and tests – all appropriate to the primary care situation – that will streamline your diagnosis and management of COPD.

*'I am sure it will become a classic in the history of COPD Care.'*

Duncan Geddes, Professor of Respiratory Medicine and Consultant Physician, Royal Brompton Hospital

### Basic Skills in Statistics    £14.99
*Adrian Cook, Gopalakrishnan Netuveli and Aziz Sheikh*

Statistics can be an intimidating subject for many students and clinicians. This concise text introduces basic concepts that underpin medical statistics and highlights the importance of statistical principles in understanding and implementing research findings in routine clinical care.

*'Packed full of useful key messages and an excellent glossary of terms, this should be an essential reference book for any budding researchers.'*

Monica Fletcher, Chief Executive, Education for Health

### Vital Asthma            £14.99
*Sue Cross and Dave Burns*

This book contains the essential information you need if you are part of the community asthma care team, whether you are a practice nurse, specialist nurse, GP, community pharmacist, physiotherapist.

*'. . . will be welcomed as a concise learning resource by those currently in asthma training, and as an update and a source of reference information by those in practice.'*

Dr Mike Thomas, FRCP, GPIAG Research Fellow, Department of General Practice, University of Aberdeen

### Vital Diabetes
THIRD EDITION            £14.99
*Dr Charles Fox and Mary MacKinnon*

This handy reference guide gives you all the back-up you need for best practice in diabetes care, and includes all the vital facts and figures about diabetes for your information and regular use, as well as providing patient and carer information sheets that you can photocopy for patients to take away with them.

*'Full of the kind of essential and up-to-date information you need to deliver the best practice in diabetes care.'*

M. Carpenter, Diabetes Grapevine

# Feedback Form

*I, the author, would welcome your comments on this book. Would you like more on some subjects and less on others? Are there additional topics which you would like to see in future editions? Please help me by marking your comments on these pages, and sending them to the publisher, post-free, at*

**Class Publishing, FREEPOST, London, W6 7BR**

| Current topics | More? | Less? |
|---|---|---|
| 1 COPD: Definition and impact | ☐ | ☐ |
| 2 Presentation, diagnosis and disease severity | ☐ | ☐ |
| 3 Stopping smoking | ☐ | ☐ |
| 4 How to manage COPD – drug therapy | ☐ | ☐ |
| 5 Pulmonary rehabilitation | ☐ | ☐ |
| 6 Oxygen therapy | ☐ | ☐ |
| 7 Living with COPD | ☐ | ☐ |
| 8 Exacerbations | ☐ | ☐ |
| 9 Managing the end of life in COPD | ☐ | ☐ |
| 10 Structuring care in general practice | ☐ | ☐ |

**Additional topics**

.................................................................................................................................

.................................................................................................................................

.................................................................................................................................

**Other comments**

.................................................................................................................................

.................................................................................................................................

.................................................................................................................................

**May we contact you?**

*Name*

*Occupation*

*Address*

*Town*                            *Postcode*

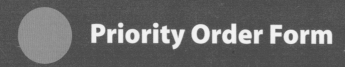

# Priority Order Form

*Cut out or photocopy this form and send it (post-free in the UK) to:*

**Class Publishing, FREEPOST 16705, Macmillan Distribution, Basingstoke RG21 6ZZ**
**Tel: 01256 302 699 / Fax: 01256 812 558**

*Please send me urgently*

| No. of copies | | Post included price per copy |
|---|---|---|
| _____ | *Vital COPD* (ISBN 1 85959 114 0) | £17.99 |
| _____ | *Chronic Obstructive Pulmonary Disease in Primary Care* (ISBN 1 85959 104 3) | £32.99 |
| _____ | *Basic Skills in Statistics* (ISBN 1 85959 101 9) | £17.99 |
| _____ | *Vital Asthma* (ISBN 1 85959 107 8) | £17.99 |
| _____ | *Vital Diabetes* (ISBN 1 85959 088 8) | £17.99 |
| | TOTAL | £_____ |

## Easy ways to pay

**1.** I enclose a cheque made payable to Class Publishing for  £_____

**2.** Please charge my    Mastercard ☐    Visa ☐    Amex ☐

*Card Number* _____  *Expiry date* _____

*Name* _____

*My address for delivery is* _____

*Town* _____

*County* _____  *Postcode* _____

*Telephone number (in case of query)* _____

*Credit card billing address (if different from above)* _____

*Town* _____

*County* _____  *Postcode* _____

*Class Publishing's guarantee: remember that if, for any reason, you are not satisfied with these books, we will refund all your money, without any questions asked. Prices and VAT rates may be altered for reasons beyond our control.*